# PRAISE FOR *THE GUTSMART PROTOCOL*

"With *The GutSMART Protocol*, Dr. Pedre has once again raised the bar and set a new standard in personalized medicine, ushering in a new era in health care!"
**—Mark Hyman, MD, *New York Times* bestselling author of *The Pegan Diet* and senior advisor, Cleveland Clinic Center for Functional Medicine**

"The smartest thing you can do is to read *The GutSMART Protocol* right now! Dr. Vincent Pedre will teach you how to finally and easily heal your gut for the ultimate upgrade in how you feel every day."
**—Dave Asprey, father of biohacking, founder of Bulletproof, and *New York Times* bestselling author**

"In the tradition of Hippocrates, *The GutSmart Protocol* emphasizes the pivotal role of gut health in the health and functionality of virtually every other organ in the human body. And gratefully, Dr. Pedre takes us beyond the science that validates this premise to deftly guide us with a program to bring about total body revitalization."
**—David Perlmutter, MD, board-certified neurologist and author of #1 *New York Times* bestseller, *Grain Brain*, and *Drop Acid***

"My fellow functional medicine practitioner, Dr. Vincent Pedre, makes the science of healing the gut easy to understand. The personalized quiz and strategies in *The GutSMART Protocol* will help you achieve that flat belly, gain more energy, manage your weight, and destress your mind and gut. A splendid common-sense approach to overall health."
**—Amy Myers, MD, *New York Times* bestselling author of *The Autoimmune Solution* and *The Thyroid Connection***

"In *The GutSMART Protocol*, Dr. Pedre bridges the science of the gut and the gut microbiome with optimal wellness and empowers readers with easy, gut-friendly recipes and adaptable meal plans. This book is an invaluable resource for anyone who is struggling with food sensitivities, sugar cravings, and weight loss resistance!"
**—JJ Virgin, *New York Times* bestselling author, founder and CEO of The Mindshare Summit**

"Incredible read! This book does an outstanding job of defining the role of gut health differently than any book I have read yet . . . while leaving very tactical and practical action steps. I can't wait to share this with my friends, family, and community."
**—Joe Mechlinski, CEO of SHIFT, *New York Times* bestselling author**

"Dr. Pedre is an incredible expert on all things gut-related. In *The GutSMART Protocol*, he deftly brings us up to speed with the latest research and helps us understand why we have to pay attention to gut health and the gut microbiome if we want to achieve optimal health. This book will be a fantastic resource for the health-conscious for years to come!"
**—Jason Wachob, founder & co-CEO, mindbodygreen**

"I love, love, love how Dr. Pedre delivers game-changing information for gut health and whole body health. It's fun, accessible, motivating, smart, doable, and science-backed! This book is no exception. Dr. Pedre, thank you for being such a bright light in gut health!"

—Dr. Kara Fitzgerald, NMD, author of *Younger You: Reduce Your Bio Age and Live Longer, Better*

"In *The GutSMART Protocol*, Dr. Pedre deftly brings us up to speed with the latest research on the gut and gut microbiome and helps us understand why we have to pay attention to them if we want to achieve optimal health for our entire body, including our thyroid. With easy, gut-friendly recipes and adaptable meal plans, he empowers readers to personalize their own gut-healing journey. This book will be an invaluable resource for anyone seeking to build the foundation of their health for years to come!"

—Izabella Wentz, PharmD, pharmacist, *New York Times* bestselling author of *Hashimoto's Protocol*

"*The GutSMART Protocol* is a thoughtfully synthesized review of the critical role that nutrition and the gut microbiome play as root causes in either driving illness or promoting wellness. Dr. Pedre clearly shows us with words and wonderful recipes how the diversity of our foods leads to the diversity and richness of our microbiome, and how that leads to the richness of our health! Follow *The GutSMART Protocol*. . . and finally enjoy the journey to health and well-being."

—Patrick Hanaway, MD, IFM Linus Pauling Award, first medical director of Cleveland Clinic Center for Functional Medicine

"Dr. Pedre's protocols on gut health have been key tools in my own health toolbox for years and so I'm thrilled that now with his new book, *The GutSMART Protocol*, these tools will be available to the millions of people worldwide suffering from gut problems and the health issues they create."

—Dr. Mariza Snyder, national bestselling author of *The Essential Oils Hormone Solution*

"Dr. Pedre has been a beacon of light in gut health education for over a decade. His work acknowledges the core essential link between gut health, human health, and our relationship to ecosystems and the natural world at large. This book promotes our potential for healing both people and the planet."

—Rob Herring, director of "The Need to GROW" and cofounder of Earth Conscious Life

"Dr. Pedre applies extensive clinical experience, scientific insight, and personal commitment to provide the most comprehensive guide to gut health yet. A must read for anyone concerned about gut health or the impact of the gut on systemic health and well-being."

—Leo Galland, MD, author of *The Allergy Solution*

"Dr. Pedre brilliantly navigates us through the fascinating but complex world of diet and the gut's influence on the body. He provides both simple and practical ways to achieve optimal health. *The GutSMART Protocol* first helps you identify your level of gut dysfunction with his highly detailed GutSMART Quiz, and then Dr. Pedre and Chef Lee Holmes provide a categorized food list, personalized meal plans, and mouth-watering recipes to aid your path to optimal gut health! SMART!"

**—Ann Louise Gittleman, Ph.D, CNS, award-winning *New York Times* bestselling author of 36 books**

"Dr. Vincent Pedre has dedicated himself to helping people get their guts healthy so they can be happy—and he drops all of his gems about the process in this book. *The GutSmart Protocol* is a great resource!"

**—Maya Shetreat, MD, author of *The Dirt Cure* and director of the Terrain Institute**

"Good health and glowing skin start in the gut! *The GutSMART Protocol* will give you a better understanding of the fascinating world of the gut microbiome, why your gut may be off balance, and how to improve it through simple diet and lifestyle changes."

**—Maria Marlowe, certified nutritionist and author of *The Clear Skin Plan***

"You can't heal your gut and body with a stressed-out mindset, and Dr. Pedre is one doctor who REALLY gets it. In *The GutSMART Protocol*, he skillfully explains why the gut-brain connection is the key to our vitality. It's why this book is a must-have solution for our collective mind-body unwellness, with its personalized approach and, yes, stress-relieving breathwork, mindfulness, and meditation exercises to bring it all home."

**—Emily Fletcher, founder of Ziva Meditation, and author of *Stress Less, Accomplish More***

"With his latest book, *The GutSMART Protocol*, Dr. Pedre is like a comforting friend who takes you by the hand and guides you step by step to help you understand the dramatic health impacts of the gut and how to create your own personalized gut-healing plan. What I love about his approach is that he's not just a medical doctor treating symptoms with drugs, he values the importance of mindfulness and stress reduction in healing the gut, body, AND your mind. This makes his book a very effective manual for healing beyond the gut."

**—Amanda Gilbert, author of *Kindness Now***

"Dr. Pedre provides readers with a simple and highly-effective path toward healthy digestion and optimal wellness. Combining his years of clinical experience with the latest science on gut health and the microbiome, *The GutSMART Protocol* equips readers with the personalized gut-healing book of the decade. What sets it apart is how Dr. Pedre delivers his wisdom with intention and heart."

**—Sachin Patel, founder of The Living Proof Institute**

# THE
# GUT**SMART**
## PROTOCOL

## Also by Vincent Pedre, MD

*HAPPY GUT:*
*The Cleansing Program to Help You Lose Weight,*
*Gain Energy, and Eliminate Pain*

# THE
# GUT**SMART**
## PROTOCOL

Revitalize Your Health, Boost Your Energy,
and Lose Weight in Just 14 Days with
Your Personalized Gut-Healing Plan

# VINCENT PEDRE, MD

## WITH LEE HOLMES, CLINICAL NUTRITIONIST

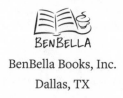

BenBella Books, Inc.
Dallas, TX

BenBella Books, Inc.
10440 N. Central Expressway
Suite 800
Dallas, TX 75231
benbellabooks.com
Send feedback to feedback@benbellabooks.com

*BenBella* is a federally registered trademark.

GutSMART® is a registered trademark of Wellness Media LLC (d/b/a Dr. Pedre Wellness).
HAPPY GUT® is a registered trademark of Wellness Media LLC (d/b/a Dr. Pedre Wellness).

Printed in the United States of America
10 9 8 7 6 5 4 3 2 1

Library of Congress Control Number: 2022044282
ISBN 9781637742556 (hardcover)
ISBN 9781637742563 (electronic)

Editing by Leah Wilson
Copyediting by Karen Wise
Proofreading by Rebecca Maines and Lisa Story
Indexing by WordCo.
Text design and composition by Aaron Edmiston
Cover design by Ty Nowicki
Food photography by Andreana Bitsis
Printed by Lake Book Manufacturing

*For Ambrose:*

*Your love, kindness, and compassion breathe through me and filter into all of my work. I hope this inspires you to see the potential within.*

*For my patients
and all the people I serve:*

*Thank you for being the inspiration behind everything that I create to help others better their health.*

# CONTENTS

# PART III. THE GUTSMART® KITCHEN

# PART IV. TURBOCHARGING YOUR RESULTS

# FOREWORD

### by David Perlmutter, MD

**While many medical conditions may involve seemingly unrelated** areas of the body, there's actually quite a bit of commonality between various conditions, at least in terms of the underlying mechanisms. One recurrent theme among all diseases is the important causative role of inflammation. Allergies, asthma, skin rashes, autoimmune diseases, diabetes, Alzheimer's disease, Parkinson's disease, coronary artery disease, and essentially every chronic degenerative condition are ultimately caused by inflammation. And as we have only recently learned, our intestinal bacteria—the gut microbiome—are hugely influential in determining the level of inflammation within our bodies.

Mechanistically, this influence begins with the health of the intestinal lining, as Dr. Vincent Pedre explains in this book. When the integrity of the gut lining is compromised, it literally opens the door to inflammation, allowing bacteria, bacterial DNA, and bacterial cell-wall components that normally reside exclusively within the intestines to leak through the intestinal lining and powerfully stimulate the immune system, leading to increased levels of the very chemicals that promote inflammation in the body. Increased permeability of the gut lining, otherwise known as "leaky gut," increases the production of inflammation-signaling chemicals and can induce damaging inflammatory changes in distant areas, including the skin, the joints, the lungs, and even the brain. Therefore, maintaining the integrity of the gut lining should be a paramount goal for each of us, equivalent to maintaining a state of health and wellness in our bodies.

As it turns out, one of the key functions of our gut bacteria is the day-to-day maintenance of this important barrier. And it's never been clearer that nurturing our gut flora *through the foods we eat* is what allows these organisms to maintain the integrity of the gut lining and thus helps us achieve lower levels of inflammation. It is this understanding that allows us to embrace the notion that our food choices are absolutely our most powerful opportunity to resist chronic degenerative conditions and live a longer and healthier life.

In the pages that follow, Dr. Pedre, with the help of clinical nutritionist and chef Lee Holmes, leverages this newly discovered connection between food choices and our health. You will learn how the foods you choose to consume, because of their influence on the health and activity of your gut organisms, ultimately influence the set point of inflammation in your body, and as such, powerfully relate to your risk for chronic degenerative disease, other inflammatory disorders, and even autoimmune conditions. Then, the prescriptive part of this text—created by a medical doctor working with a nutritionist/chef—will give you the tools to reestablish a meaningful and salubrious relationship with the 100 trillion bacteria that not only live within you, but are highly influential in determining your health destiny. Dr. Pedre first helps you identify your level of gut dysfunction with his highly detailed GutSMART Quiz, which determines your inflammation burden, then provides specific meal plans to support you on your gut-healing journey, regardless of where on that journey you are.

Like his first book, *Happy Gut*, Dr. Pedre's latest book is a rich amalgam of his clinical wisdom, much of it gained from helping patients with gut issues and chronic, gut-related degenerative health problems achieve optimal health. It is a must for anyone looking to build a foundation of gut health to support their total wellness.

**David Perlmutter, MD**
*New York Times* bestselling author of *Grain Brain*

# WHERE DISEASE BEGINS

> *"Something there is that doesn't love a wall . . .*
> *And makes gaps even two can pass abreast."*
>
> —Robert Frost

**Imagine your body as an ancient city surrounded by a wall. The** wall protects the city by keeping out invaders and other unfriendly visitors. The city needs to trade, however, and to allow goods to enter through the city walls. It cannot be completely isolated. So there are entrances throughout that allow for the controlled flow of goods, food, and water. The city also has an army to monitor the activity along the wall, making sure no unwanted trespassers enter through the barricades. In effect, this ancient city must balance interacting with the outside world with the protection of its borders.

Such a wall would be subject to the disruptive effects of the environment, and to being chipped away at by foes seeking to sneak in without being seen. Therefore, the wall would need to be maintained. It would need to be repaired constantly with new bricks and cement to preserve its integrity over time. If a sudden explosion ever created a hole in the wall, it would be met by skilled soldiers trained to prevent an invasion. Any breaches would lead to a battle—one that would either be resolved quickly or, if the enemy were strong enough to inflict continuing damage on the protected city while resisting a counterattack, persist indefinitely.

That city wall is the inner lining of your digestive tract. When healthy, it acts as a semipermeable membrane that selectively allows nutrients, minerals, and other products of digestion into the rest of your body while keeping out dangerous pathogens. Your army is the team of white blood cells that inhabits and monitors the entire length of your gastrointestinal (GI) tract—sampling everything coming through like border patrol agents at a checkpoint and making sure that it is not a foe trying to sneak in.

When all is well, there are no breaches in the wall and no major battles being waged. However, the sad truth is we are in the middle of an epidemic of GI disease that is growing exponentially, putting that wall (our inner gut lining) under constant attack. The pooled prevalence rates of irritable bowel syndrome (IBS) in eighty study populations, representing a total of 260,960 subjects across all continents, was 11.2 percent, with no rate lower than 7 percent. Based on an estimated world population of 8 billion (as of November 2022[1]), this suggests there are a staggering *896 million individuals* suffering from IBS worldwide. So it's no wonder that, over the last several decades, gut-related disorders have skyrocketed[2]—something I have witnessed firsthand in my own medical practice.

Gut disorders are an unspoken source of the epidemic of unwellness that plagues modern society. People with gut dysfunction tend to have higher rates of mood disorders, anxiety, depression, mental fog, fatigue, and poor focus. It not only affects the individual; it affects their entire social network. When a person suffers this way, the people around them suffer as well. Whenever a loved one is unwell, it weighs upon those closest to them. No person is an island unto themselves when it comes to chronic illness.

Why have gut and gut-related disorders become such an epidemic? Over the last hundred years, there have been significant changes in the way we live and eat that have led to the disruption of the delicate homeostasis found within the gut ecosystem. The list of gut disruptors is long and continues to grow. It includes:

- poor diet (the Standard American Diet, or SAD, which is unfortunately being exported worldwide), including excessive consumption of processed foods

- food additives used by the food industry to create unnatural textures and flavors
- exaggerated hygiene (excess cleanliness)
- lack of contact with soil and livestock
- inadequate hydration or dehydration
- infections (bacteria, yeast, and/or parasites)
- medications (antibiotics, anti-inflammatories, oral contraceptive pills)
- hormone-disrupting chemicals (BPA, fire retardants, nonstick cookware) and toxins (heavy metals, mold, pesticides, GMOs)
- prolonged, unrelenting stress

Exposure to these disruptors wreaks havoc on the gut: vagal nerve dysfunction (which affects the heart, lungs, and digestive tract), inadequate digestive enzyme production, low stomach acid, deficient bile acids/gallbladder dysfunction, disrupted and imbalanced microbial ecology (lack of good gut "bugs"), impaired intestinal permeability (that is, leaky gut), and impaired intestinal motility. The result is a sad gut, characterized by bloating, indigestion, heartburn, diarrhea, constipation, and/or abdominal pain. And a sad gut can then lead to a "sad body" and sad mind. But that's only the tip of the iceberg.

The problems heavily impacted by this gut disruption epidemic are more far-reaching than people realize because **you don't even have to suffer from any gut symptoms to have a gut-related disorder**. For many people, the signals of poor gut health don't come from their gut but from other parts of their body. Their joints may ache, their bodies feel tired, and their brains feel foggy—all while their gut, the source of it all, sits silently, seemingly innocently, on the sidelines.

These gut-related signals can come in the form of . . .

## Systemic conditions
- Allergies
- Asthma
- Autoimmune disease
- Chronic fatigue
- Joint pain (osteoarthritis)
- Muscle aches

## Skin issues

- Acne
- Eczema
- Hives
- Psoriasis
- Rosacea

## Neurological conditions

- Anxiety
- Attention-Deficit Hyperactivity Disorder (ADHD)
- Autism
- Dementia
- Mental fog
- Migraines
- Neurological diseases (Parkinson's, Alzheimer's)

. . . and we're learning more connections between the gut and disease every day.

Simply put, **there is no system left untouched by the state of your gut**. And that means improving your health requires a *whole gut-body-mind approach*—which is exactly what this book provides.

The dietary recommendations and stress-reduction techniques I describe in the coming chapters, which are simple but incredibly powerful, have tremendous potential to balance your gut flora and transform your health. With tried-and-true strategies that have already helped thousands of people overcome gut issues worldwide, I show you the key interventions that will improve the diversity of your gut microbiota to help you feel great and prevent or even reverse disease—and even lose weight in the process.[3]

Part I of *The GutSMART Protocol* is meant to lay the foundation, filling in any gaps in your knowledge about how gut health relates to the rest of your body and brain. (If you read my previous book, *Happy Gut*, you'll recognize the broad strokes, but I've included the latest science and most up-to-date knowledge about the gut and gut microbiome from the many new studies that have been published since then.) In chapter 1, "It Starts with the Gut," we explore the gut as the foundation of health, looking at how microbial imbalances known as *dysbiosis* can lead to a compromised gut barrier (aka "leaky gut syndrome"), which opens up the floodgates of inflammation—the root cause of every chronic, degenerative disease. In chapter 2, "Fix Your Gut, Fix Your Body," we continue to explore the effects of leaky gut on the whole body, including the connections between the gut and your skin, energy, metabolism, and brain. By allowing all sorts of inflammatory molecules—including the worst of them, *endotoxin*—to enter your body and trigger inflammation everywhere, including in your brain, leaky gut is disclosed as the silent scourge of the unwell, including those suffering from metabolic derangements that can lead to weight gain.[4]

In chapter 3, "The Microbiome Revolution," I reveal an updated view of how the world of bacteria living symbiotically within you—your *gut microbiome*—affects your health. The microbiome is a very complex symbiotic system that we are still learning about, and the latest research suggests it is even more in control of your well-being than we knew. Imbalance in the gut flora—the dysbiosis mentioned above—not only wreaks havoc in your digestive system, but also leads to chronic inflammation and chronic activation of the immune system, becoming the kindling wood for the fires of chronic degenerative conditions throughout the body.

The modern-life stressors that lead to dysbiosis are explored in chapters 4 and 5, including antibiotics, environmental toxins and pesticides, GMOs (from glyphosate sprayed on our biggest crops—wheat, corn, and soy), sleep deprivation, excessive hygiene, and chronic stress. But nothing creates quite the whammy against gut health as poor diet—which is why, after laying down the foundation, we turn our attention to the foods we should eat and to creating a personalized plan that will revolutionize your gut health for whole body-mind wellness.

In Part II, it's time to get GutSMART! In chapter 6, you'll use the GutSMART Quiz to determine your level of gut dysfunction (Severe, Moderate, or Mild). Your GutSMART Score will help you determine the right place to begin your food-based, gut-healing journey. From there, you will be guided through the GutSMART Protocol, appropriately tailored to your individual needs. This isn't a one-size-fits-all diet protocol. It's designed to take your current level of gut dysfunction into account, as well as be easy to modify based on your personal food preferences and sensitivities.

Chapter 7 outlines the 14-Day GutSMART Protocol—your first step to healing your gut and balancing your gut microbiome, so you can get started feeling great (and, if it's one of your goals, losing weight) as soon as possible! In it, I reveal the five gut superfoods that should be part of any gut-healing program. And I introduce the three types of intuitive eating as one of the most important skills to develop as you embark on your gut restoration journey.

From there, we jump to the GutSMART Kitchen, where chef and clinical nutritionist Lee Holmes and I have teamed up to engineer the right meal plan for your GutSMART type. Chapter 8 presents three suggested 14-day meal plans using recipes in the book, one for Mild gut dysfunction, one for Moderate, and one for Severe. You can follow these meal plans exactly, or mix and match according to my GutSMART Protocol guidelines. (We know how busy you are, and wanted to do the food and prep thinking for you so you can simply relax and follow the plan.) Or you can just use them as a source of inspiration to see what it looks like to eat right while healing your gut. I provide general guidance as well to help you when eating out.

Since the GutSMART Protocol is mostly dairy-free for those who get a Moderate or Severe score on the GutSMART Quiz, we'll also guide you on the basics of making your own nut milks, free of preservatives and additives and gut-friendlier than the store-bought versions. These nut milks will become a base for many other recipes. For vegetarians or vegans who rely on beans as their major source of protein but need to heal their guts, I also explain how to make beans more gut-friendly.

Speaking of recipes . . . chapter 9 is my favorite! It's full of all sorts of gut-friendly recipes to give you plenty of options, whether you are vegan, vegetarian, paleo-minded, pescatarian, or something in between. From smoothies, juices, and mocktails to nourishing soups, savory salads, and delicious entrees for all eating preferences, we're sure to have a recipe you'll want to make over and over for yourself and share with family and friends. We also include side dishes, fermented delights, and guilt-free desserts you can eat to your heart's desire.

The goal of the GutSMART Protocol is to teach you how to live with a happy gut for life, free of the sorts of problems an unhappy gut can create. Part IV of the book is all about *turbocharging your results* through breathwork and meditation. You can skip ahead and read this part before you start the GutSMART Protocol or wait to turn your attention here once you have your GutSMART Score and feel you have a good grasp of the protocol. Chapter 10 will teach you how to harness the power of your vagus nerve through activation techniques like deep, diaphragmatic breathing so you can live in greater digestive harmony. In chapter 11, I team up with breathwork experts to bring you breathing exercises that help improve the functioning of your gut and relax your nervous system. We take this a step further in chapter 12, "The Zen Gut," by asking two world-leading meditation experts to teach us their best meditations for a healthy, calm digestive system and happy mind. And I end it with my very own Gut-Love Meditation—a reworking of the well-known Tibetan Buddhist loving-compassion meditation technique.

Finally, I talk about what's next: how to live a GutSMART life going forward. The 14-Day GutSMART Protocol is just the beginning, meant to set the wheels of wellness in motion in the right direction so you can live your best life yet, free of gut concerns—and more! You won't want to miss my FREE GIVEAWAY (page 288), which will help reinforce a lot of what you've learned in this book and continue to inspire you to live a happy gut life.

For those who want to go deeper, in the Appendix, I explain how you can use the 14-Day GutSMART Protocol as a springboard to dive into my more intensive program for gut-healing—the HAPPY GUT® Reboot: 28-Day  Cleanse, featured in my first book, *Happy Gut: The Cleansing Program to Help You Lose Weight, Gain Energy, and Eliminate Pain*—and include a ***special offer*** for readers of this book. It's an opportunity to deepen your results or resolve gut-related symptoms that were not completely addressed by the Gut-SMART Protocol.

This book is only the beginning of the deep healing that is waiting for you and your gut! It's time to revitalize your health, boost your energy, and lose weight in just 14 days with your personalized gut-healing plan, so you can feel the best you've felt in years.

All it takes is one word: *commitment!* And that commitment is not just to following the GutSMART Protocol, but to becoming the best version of *YOU*. Let the best of you shine bright by healing from the inside out. It's not just a diet, it's the springboard for a new lifestyle.

But before we embark on this journey together, let me share my story, along with that of chef and clinical nutritionist Lee Holmes, so you can understand why I wrote this book, why I'm so passionate about helping others heal their gut-related health issues, and why Lee was the perfect choice to create the gut-healing recipes you'll soon be enjoying!

# OUR GUT-HEALING JOURNEYS

## DR. PEDRE'S GUT-HEALING JOURNEY

The reason I'm here today, writing this book, is because I struggled with gut health issues for the greater part of my life—from early childhood all the way into my mid-thirties. And I can't bear seeing others suffering for as long as I did without a solution. For the longest time, I (and before that, my parents) thought my upset stomach and abdominal pain, which ranged from moderate to severe, had everything to do with something internal (like the constipation I suffered from as a preteen) and nothing to do with anything external (the foods I ate, the antibiotics I had repeatedly been on, and the stress that plagued me as a type A overachieving child and teenager).

I wish I could say that healing my gut was easy—that it only took meeting the right doctor who said just the right things to turn my gut health around. But instead of making my gut-related issues better, doctors often made them worse. And since no one gave my gut issues serious consideration (other than trying to treat symptoms, which sometimes helped and sometimes did not), I came to think of upset stomachs, bloating, gas, and abdominal pain as part of my operating system—a background program running on the computer hard drive of my life. I considered it my "normal." Can you relate?

When I was a child, I had a "nervous stomach." I used to play the piano, and whenever I had a recital or competition, I felt like I had a swarm of butterflies doing somersaults inside my belly as I anticipated that moment I would have to walk on stage. My stomach would feel so awful that I couldn't eat in the hours leading up to a performance to keep myself from feeling sick and nauseous.

But the problems weren't confined to my belly. I caught so many upper respiratory infections, which often turned into sinusitis or bronchitis, that my pediatrician was concerned about my immune system. He prescribed a multivitamin, thinking it would strengthen my defenses. It didn't work. This was back in the 1980s, before we understood that the gut is the gateway to our immunity and that the foods we eat can affect how our immune systems function. The daily sugary wheat cereals with milk for breakfast and afterschool fast-food milkshakes my mom would take me to get on the way home were, in addition to giving me a sad gut, weakening my immune system. They were also making me feel tired, and left me foggy-headed, often for hours, because—as I discovered years later—I had become sensitive to dairy. Like most families at the time, we thought that "milk does the body good," but it did my body *bad*.

It wasn't until I was in medical school in my early twenties, when out of practicality I cut out cereal with milk for breakfast, that I stopped getting sick all the time. I simply didn't have the time to sit down and eat breakfast when I had to rush out the door to early morning classes. All those years, I had believed, like most of us do, that milk was good for me. When I made the connection between avoiding milk and getting fewer colds or sinus infections, I had my first "Eureka!" moment: Diet clearly played a major role in how my body felt and how my immune system behaved. Little did I know, that was the beginning of a shift in my perspective on what creates holistic wellness that would bring me here today, speaking to you about how diet affects the gut and, honestly, everything about your health.

While in medical school, because of the previous damage to my gut, I struggled with how I couldn't eat the same foods my fellow doctors-to-be could without suffering secondary consequences, like having to suddenly run to the bathroom. And as I embarked on my own journey to creating a happy gut, it took me almost another decade of trial and error to fully grasp the best way to eat for my own gut and body, while learning what worked for other guts and bodies. By making a few additional changes in my diet, including adding more healthy fats, I felt better than I ever had before. However, I still wasn't in the clear.

You see, what had begun as a nervous stomach in my childhood turned into irritable bowel syndrome (IBS) by my mid- to late twenties. By then, I had discovered meditation and had learned to calm my nerves through breathing techniques (like the ones in chapter 11), but stress was still doing a number on my gut. And sure, I wasn't getting as many upper respiratory infections, but I was still eating foods that were harming my gut.

It wasn't until I discovered functional medicine that I was able to rewrite my entire story, from the beginning to the present, in a way that made my health issues make sense. I realized the twenty-plus rounds of antibiotics I had been on as a child had destroyed my gut microbiome, decimating its health-promoting diversity. As a result, I'd ended up with a leaky gut, which then led me to develop sensitivities to the top foods in the diet of almost every teenager: wheat (gluten) and dairy. I had literally been poisoning my gut—and through it, my entire body—for decades.

So, I embarked on a major project—healing my gut. Honestly, I had no idea if it was going to work. The concept of the gut microbiome seemed like something from a sci-fi movie. Little bacteria in our guts seriously exerted that much power over us?! And yet, I started a gut-healing regimen with absolute faith, trusting that it would take some time before I noticed the results. I made changes in my diet by eating organic, adding in fermented foods, and avoiding gluten and dairy, along with a list of other foods I had discovered I was sensitive to.

Within the first two weeks, I already noticed a difference in my digestion. It was quieter and less painful, and my bowel movements were better formed. What a relief! Had those things not improved, I would have been disheartened; they were the results I was expecting. What was unexpected was the increase in my energy levels, mental clarity, and ability to stay sharp all the way to the end of a ten- to twelve-hour workday.

Wow! By working on my gut health, I not only improved how my gut functioned, but also boosted my productivity at work, overcame the cloud of fatigue that had engulfed me (and that I attributed solely to my long work hours), and sharpened my focus. I knew I was on to something, and so I started really zeroing in on my patients' gut health issues, working to improve them. The results were extraordinary! Not only did their gut health improve, but other long-standing health issues magically and unexpectedly disappeared. My patients were pleasantly surprised—and so was I!

By healing my gut, not only did I give myself another lease on life (I was already starting to feel old and worn-down by my mid-thirties), but I was able to shatter my long-held belief that my gut health issues were a lifelong sentence. They weren't! And they don't have to be for you, either. I want to give you a new lease on life as well!

Since the publishing of my first book, *Happy Gut*, I have helped thousands of people around the globe improve their health by first helping them improve the foundation for all wellness—their digestive system (aka "the gut"). And I wanted to make my protocols even more accessible and easier for as many people as possible. That's why I sat down to write this book. I've learned so much since *Happy Gut* that I'm excited to share with you to help you quickly and effectively forge a path from a sad gut inside a sad body, plagued by a sad mind, to a happy gut in a happy body with a happy mind.

My "new normal" is digestive harmony no matter what. I can even enjoy eating out again as much as eating at home, because I know the right food choices to make. I've made it into my lifestyle, not just a diet. And I wish all of this for you, as well. I hope my gut-healing journey inspires you to see through the fog of whatever chronic gut and gut-related health issues you have been dealing with to the possibility of a healthier, happier life for yourself. There is a light at the end of the tunnel of your gut-related disturbances—and *The GutSMART Protocol* is your roadmap to getting there.

## CHEF LEE HOLMES'S GUT-HEALING JOURNEY

Hi, I'm Lee Holmes, a clinical nutritionist, whole-food chef, and yoga and meditation teacher. A number of years ago, I was enjoying a fast-paced career with ABC in Sydney, Australia, helping to promote acts like the Wiggles, when I suddenly became ill.

I felt so unwell I could scarcely haul myself out of bed and go to work. At first, I chalked it up to life without a pause button; I was a busy, working single parent, and I was used to feeling tired. But this felt different. What I didn't realize back then was that I would be among the one in twenty people in Australia diagnosed with autoimmune diseases—startlingly, most of them women. My body's immune system had somehow gone haywire and turned on itself; my entire body was covered with mystery hives and I was leaving clumps of hair on my pillow.

When it first started, I went to specialists, hoping to figure out the underlying cause. I was later shocked to find out that autoimmune diseases are tied to gut health. My gut had been a weak point for most of my life, but now it was affecting so much more than just my digestion. My symptoms were as pronounced as they were sudden, and I hardly recognized myself. I was dealing with serious brain fog, aches and pains, and chronic fatigue, and my weight quickly plummeted to 42 kilograms (around 92 pounds).

After months of seeing specialist after specialist, and after lots of eye-rolling, head-nodding, and to-ing and fro-ing, I was diagnosed with nonspecific autoimmune disease and fibromyalgia.

During this time, I was in and out of hospitals and being given steroids, antibiotics, and immunosuppressant drugs, which only made me feel worse because of their multiple side effects. It got to the point where I couldn't differentiate between the side effects of the medication and the symptoms of my condition. Fortunately, I got my doctors to agree to allow me to wean myself off the medication if I started to improve with dietary changes.

I simplified my diet, lessening the number of triggers like food additives, MSG, and highly processed foods, and immediately saw a big improvement in my health: My puffiness subsided, my hives disappeared, and my energy levels improved.

Learning the impact the gut has on the immune system and the links between diet, digestion, and improved immunity was earth-shattering. At a young age, I had been placed on six consecutive rounds of antibiotics for chronic interstitial cystitis; this was the beginning of my health decline, though it wasn't until I was in my forties that the majority of my problems started.

With my newfound energy and interest in learning more about the connections between my diet, gut health, and the symptoms I was experiencing, I researched the medicinal capabilities of ingredients and how they could be used to improve health. I started creating recipes in my kitchen, planting the seeds that became the roots of my blog, superchargedfood.com. I've gone on to publish nine bestselling books featuring easy, nutritious recipes that not only taste delicious and are simple to make but also help you feel amazing. My desire was, and still is, to make healthy eating delicious, simple, and gut-friendly for everyone.

When Dr. Pedre asked me to be part of this book, I jumped at the chance. We are kindred spirits on opposite sides of the world, and I have loved every moment of creating gut-friendly recipes based on his proven GutSMART principles. As a clinical nutritionist, I truly believe that a healthy gut is critical for a healthy body, no matter what your current level of health is. The recipes I've put together will help motivate you to not only eat more gut-friendly foods, but also feel at home in the kitchen. My goal in contributing to *The GutSMART Protocol* is simple: to inspire you to create easy and tasty meals that will satisfy your appetite and provide the gut-healing, nutritional benefits you need to thrive.

# PART I
# BUILDING THE
# FOUNDATION

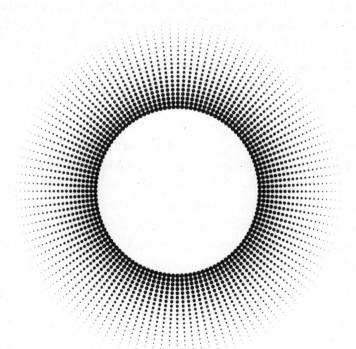

# Chapter 1

# IT STARTS WITH THE GUT

> *"When solving problems, dig at the roots instead of just hacking at the leaves."*
>
> —Anthony J. D'Angelo
>
> (author and founder of the Inspiration Book Series)

**Now that you're ready to begin your healing journey, let's get a few** things out of the way . . .

First, I want to congratulate you. (*For what, Dr. Pedre? I haven't done anything yet.*) The way I see it, your decision to pick up this book is a major victory. You're choosing to reclaim your health and get to the bottom of whatever gut-related health issues you're dealing with, and in my experience, that is no easy feat.

Second, you should know that this book isn't like any other book on gut health that you've read (my previous book included!), because it's designed to be personalized for your needs . . . and yes, I did that on purpose.

You see, I've been working in the medical field for over two decades, and too often, I come across books that are one of the following (or a combination of the three):

1.  **Not actionable**—They don't give you concrete steps or advice.

2. **Impractical**—If they do recommend concrete steps or advice, what they want you to do is either not feasible or too complicated.

3. **Too general**—The recommendations aren't personalized for you.

Think about it: How many times have you read an article about wellness or a health book and then thought, *Okay, now what?* or worse, *Oh, I can't do that.* That experience is frustrating and discouraging, especially when you're ready and eager to make a change.

After all, what's the point of having knowledge if you don't know what to do with it? When I set out to write *The GutSMART Protocol*, I wanted to make it as accessible and doable for anyone who reads it as it is comprehensive. I wanted to create plans and instructions that you can immediately put to use while tailoring my recommendations to fit your individual needs in a personalized way that most books don't offer, all while providing the research to back it all up.

<u>To be clear</u>: This book is not a "one size fits all" solution. Instead, after it gives you the foundation of knowledge you need upfront, you'll use the GutSMART Quiz to determine where you are in your gut-healing journey and what plan will be the best fit for you. Once you figure out which of three categories your gut dysfunction falls into—Mild (occasional symptoms), Moderate (intermittent symptoms), or Severe (acute or chronic symptoms)—I'll walk you through an individualized plan aimed at healing your gut. The best part? You can take the GutSMART Quiz more than once (don't worry, I have a downloadable digital version for you at **gutsmartprotocol. com/quiz**) and sequentially stack the plans based on your evolving quiz score. This way, you can track the progress of your gut-healing journey, while always having an individualized plan to help you along. Whatever gut issues you're dealing with, this book is here to guide you, like a friend taking you home.

My hope is that you'll move through this book efficiently and effectively—taking it all in, familiarizing yourself with the information, and then converting that information into action. That said, this book will bring up a lot of thoughts, questions, and feelings (of hope, maybe concern, and even discomfort), but it's all in the interest of helping you live your best life with the most optimal health—the health that starts in your gut.

So, let's roll up our sleeves and get to work.

## A LITTLE BIT ABOUT MY APPROACH

The majority of people in the United States (and even worldwide) are accustomed to the Western model of care—they have checkups once a year, sprinkled with sick visits where they might be prescribed antibiotics, and in between these visits refill prescriptions that suppress the symptoms they're experiencing but don't necessarily address the root cause of those symptoms.

I am a board-certified internist, and I have spent years studying Western medicine, but my approach to health—especially gut health—is instead rooted in **functional medicine**. In functional medicine, a single "disease" may be the result of a combination of factors, and functional medicine's practice is all about uncovering the underlying causes of that disease rather than just treating symptoms. The goal is to figure out what's going wrong in the body that's causing these symptoms to appear—and from there, to treat not just the symptoms, but also the cause with diet, nutrition, lifestyle changes, mindfulness practices, and supplements if indicated.

One of my favorite metaphors for describing the difference between the Western medicine model and functional medicine involves a sick tree. When a tree's

## SICK TREE ANALOGY
WESTERN MEDICINE vs. FUNCTIONAL MEDICINE

WESTERN MEDICINE

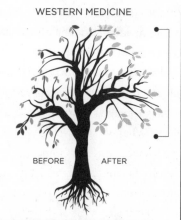

BEFORE          AFTER

FUNCTIONAL MEDICINE

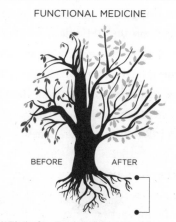

BEFORE          AFTER

In the Western medicine model, when a tree is sick and the leaves look brown and diseased, we "cure" the tree by painting the leaves green—the equivalent of giving someone a medication to treat a symptom instead of figuring out the actual cause and addressing it.

With the functional medicine approach, when a tree is sick and the leaves look limp, we don't treat the leaves. Instead, we look at the roots and fix the problem at its source. This is the equivalent of healing the gut—the body's "root system"—to heal the body.

leaves look brown and diseased, you don't cure the tree by painting the leaves green. Instead, you look at the roots and fix the problem at its source. Think of your digestive system as the roots of a tree—your gut is the root system of your body. When things go wrong on the surface, you've got to look at the roots to fix what's happening in the leaves. Painting the leaves green is the equivalent of giving someone a medication to treat a symptom instead of figuring out its cause and addressing it.

As you read through this book, rest assured that my goal is to help you heal what's been harmed, not just mask your symptoms—to treat the roots of your tree (your disease's underlying cause or causes) to make your branches and leaves (your body and brain) bright and healthy again. And for the majority of people, the root cause of their health issues lies within the gut.

# A BRIEF OVERVIEW OF THE GUT

We can talk about the gut all day, but if you aren't familiar with its purpose and function, most of what I say in this book won't make sense. So, let's start on a simple, foundational level. What is the gut, and why does it matter?

### Three Fundamental Truths about Your Gut

The term **gut** refers to your digestive system, aka your gastrointestinal (GI) tract. The primary organs we think of as being involved in digestion include the mouth, esophagus, stomach, small intestine, liver, pancreas, and large intestine. As you make your way through this chapter, you'll quickly see it's much more complex than that, but to begin, I want to share with you three fundamental truths about the gut. There's no need to commit them to memory—you'll see these ideas resurface throughout the book!

1.  *Your gut harbors the most complex ecosystem on the planet.* The human body is like an **ecosystem** (a singular environment that serves as the home for multiple living organisms), and the gut itself is an ecosystem within that ecosystem. Studies have shown time and time again how deeply complex the gut is. It contains trillions of microbes (single-celled organisms ranging from bacteria to yeast to parasites), without which, one could argue, we wouldn't be able to survive.

There are an estimated **100 trillion bacteria living in our guts, composed of an estimated 500 to 1000 species,** which together make up our gut microbiota.[1] To put this number in perspective, there are only 226,000 identified marine species in the ocean, with researchers estimating that there could be as many as 2 million marine species total globally.[2] To zoom out even further, scientists estimate that there are about 8.7 million species on Earth, including plants and animals.[3] That means **there are over 11 million times more individual microbes in the gut than there are total species on the planet.** I know it's hard to fathom, but it's true.

I'll teach you everything you need to know about the microbiome in chapter 3, but for now, remember that the gut is home to trillions of microbes that play an essential, symbiotic role in our overall health.

2.   *Your gut is connected to every system in your body.* Believe it or not, your gut is the epicenter of all bodily processes and systems. This isn't something we're taught in health class or during our annual checkups, so this idea tends to shock people. There isn't much (if anything) in your body that is unaffected by your gut. The gut plays a role in everything from your mental health and immunity to your weight, skin health, energy levels, and so much more. That is why having a healthy gut (including a healthy gut microbiome) is so important for enjoying optimal health.

3.   *Your gut is the cornerstone of your health.* This is one of several metaphors I'll return to throughout this book. If you've never heard of a cornerstone, it's essentially the starting point of construction for a structure—the first stone laid down in a building foundation. Since all the other stones will be set in relation to this stone, its placement determines how the rest of the building will be constructed. In essence, it is the single most important part of any construction project and what allows a building to withstand the test of time.

I often call the gut the "cornerstone of your health" because everything else that happens in our body is in many ways dependent on the gut's ability to absorb nutrients and keep out bad things. Thus, by strengthening your gut, you are laying the cornerstone for a solid foundation from which to build your health and wellness.

Now, let's talk about what the gut can really do.

## THE POWER OF THE GUT

I named this chapter "It Starts with the Gut," but what does that actually mean?

To me, it means that your gut is where you have to begin when it comes to healing your body, starting from the inside out. It's where we receive all of our nourishment. And it's critical and foundational for creating total wellness in the body—whether it's brain health, mental health, skin health, or heart health, every part of your body depends on a healthy gut and a healthy gut microbiome. "It Starts with the Gut" also means that, in many cases, underlying health issues, disorders, and conditions can be traced back to the gut.

That's right—the gut holds much more power than you realize, and there's a growing body of evidence to prove it. Two foundational concepts you need to know from the get-go to understand what makes for a healthy gut are **dysbiosis** and **leaky gut**.

## WHAT IS THIS THING CALLED DYSBIOSIS?

**Dysbiosis** is an imbalance between favorable and unfavorable microorganisms in the gut that tips the scales towards the unfavorable ones. There are multiple potential types of dysbiosis: an excess of bad bacteria, of yeast, of parasites, or of worms, or a combination of any of these. For example, yeast overgrowth in the gut (often referred to as *candida*) is a type of dysbiosis. The main causes of dysbiosis include the regular consumption of processed foods, exposure to pesticides, antibiotic use, OTC medications (like NSAIDs), and the modern-life stressors that we encounter on a daily basis.

*Dysbiosis* is the opposite of symbiosis: It means "living out of harmony." In other words, when you have a dysbiosis, the balance of good and bad gut bacteria, yeast, or even parasites has shifted; your bad gut bacteria, yeast, and/or parasites have taken over and are throwing an unwelcome party. Dysbiosis can happen anywhere there is a microbiome, on or inside the body: the skin, airways, sinuses, vaginal canal, and, of course, the gut.

For simplicity and for the purposes of this book, when I say "dysbiosis," I am referring to an overgrowth of bad bacteria in the gut (which could or could not be accompanied by a yeast imbalance or even parasites). Dysbiosis of the gut micro-biome has been associated with a large number of health problems and found to be a major contributing cause of metabolic, immunological, and developmental disorders, as well as increased susceptibility to infectious diseases of the digestive system (like parasites).[4] Dysbiosis tends to cause excessive gas, bloating, constipa-tion, diarrhea, indigestion, and abdominal pain, but can also be the cause of symp-toms seemingly unrelated to the gut, such as mental fog, fatigue, muscle aches, and joint inflammation.

This is what makes specific types of dysbiosis so tricky to diagnose: Their symp-toms are nonspecific (meaning, they don't just cause obvious "stomach issues") and can appear in the background of a variety of conditions. In addition to the array of gut symptoms mentioned above that can occur over time (including that "stuffed" feeling after meals!), dysbiosis symptoms can also include rashes, hives, eczema, asthma, metabolic syndrome, numbness in the hands and feet, and joint pain.

*Do any of those sound like you?*

Dysbiosis is the beginning of a downward spiral for your gut. Without proper treatment, it can eventually lead to problems like *increased intestinal permeability*, or what we call *"leaky gut,"* where partially digested food proteins, bacteria, yeast, and toxins that are not intended to get through your gut wall do, activating your immune system and turning on inflammatory signals that send your health into a nosedive.

As you'll see in upcoming chapters, dysbiosis has become a huge problem for the majority of people on this planet. Unlike food poisoning or traveler's diarrhea—which are more sudden and acute forms of dysbiosis (that is, they can be pretty dramatic, but also easily treatable)—this type of dysbiosis is chronic, subtle, and not usually amenable to a "quick fix." It evolves over time and can be present **for months or even years** before you take notice, even as it wreaks havoc inside your body. For many people, the signs and symptoms of dysbiosis become part of their "normal" as they consult Western doctors for ways to deal with the symptoms of other disorders (like autoimmune and inflammatory diseases). As a "solution," they're given Band-Aid remedies that don't address the root cause.

For many years, this was true for me. Growing up with irritable bowel syn-drome (IBS), taking over-the-counter remedies for heartburn and upset stomachs, and suffering from food sensitivities, a weakened immune system, low energy, and allergies, I came to believe this was my normal. It wasn't. As I shared previously in my gut-healing journey (page 8), the root of everything I was dealing with, I discovered over two decades later, was a leaky gut.

# INCREASED INTESTINAL PERMEABILITY (AKA "LEAKY GUT SYNDROME")

**Increased intestinal permeability**, or **leaky gut**, refers to an impairment of the semipermeable barrier between the food and bugs inside the intestines and the rest of the body, which as a result lets more through than it should. When you develop a leaky gut—which can occur as a result of any number of different causes (see "Healthy Gut vs. Leaky Gut")—the connections between the cells that line your intestinal wall and help keep that barrier sealed (known as **tight junctions**) become looser, allowing larger molecules like partially digested food proteins, bacteria, bacterial DNA, yeast, and even parasites to pass through your gut wall. Right on the other side of the inner gut lining is an area called the **lamina propria**. Think of this as the "neutral zone" between two oppositional countries bordering each other—except, in this case, it's the neutral zone between you and any bad bugs[‡] in your gut.

Within the *lamina propria*, and in the lymphatic system that runs throughout the gut lining, are patrolling white blood cells, monitoring and surveying everything coming through that one-cell-layer-thick gut lining. When the tightly bound connections between intestinal cells are relaxed and become "leaky," allowing undesirable bugs, toxins, and incompletely digested proteins to slip through into the lamina propria (that neutral zone), your immune cells pounce on what they see as potential threats, ***triggering an inflammation response.***[5]

---

[‡] There is always a subset of "bad bugs" in the gut, believed to comprise 10–15 percent of the gut microbiome in healthy individuals. It's believed that they do play some sort of yet-to-be-discovered regulatory role, but only when they are present in the right amounts.

## HEALTHY GUT vs. LEAKY GUT
How a Healthy Gut Becomes a Leaky Gut

A healthy gut keeps pathogens and toxins out. In a leaky gut, the tight junctions loosen up, allowing undigested food particles, toxins, and pathogenic bacteria, yeast, or parasites to get through the gut barrier and activate the immune system, causing inflammation and food sensitivities. Gluten, in particular, has been shown to increase gut permeability not only in people with celiac disease or gluten sensitivity, but also in normal individuals.

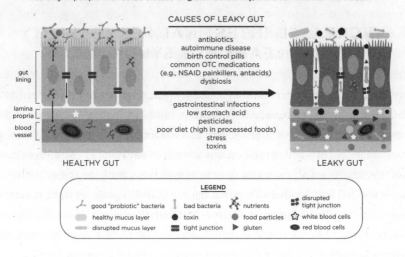

CAUSES OF LEAKY GUT

antibiotics
autoimmune disease
birth control pills
common OTC medications
(e.g., NSAID painkillers, antacids)
dysbiosis

gastrointestinal infections
low stomach acid
pesticides
poor diet (high in processed foods)
stress
toxins

gut lining

lamina propria

blood vessel

HEALTHY GUT

LEAKY GUT

**LEGEND**

| | | |
|---|---|---|
| good "probiotic" bacteria | bad bacteria | nutrients | disrupted tight junction |
| healthy mucus layer | toxin | food particles | white blood cells |
| disrupted mucus layer | tight junction | gluten | red blood cells |

Inflammation is at the root of every disease in the body. And the gut is your biggest potential source of inflammation.

# LEAKY GUT, CHRONIC INFLAMMATION & DISEASE

I can't emphasize this enough: Chronic inflammation caused by an immune system on overdrive is the major driver of every disease. This is particularly true for inflammatory bowel diseases (IBDs), such as Crohn's and ulcerative colitis, which can then affect other parts of the body, and can also be true in gut imbalances such as small intestinal bacterial overgrowth (SIBO) and yeast overgrowth (Candida) that lead to other systemic inflammatory symptoms.

Even irritable bowel syndrome (IBS),[‡] which was previously believed to impact *only* the gut, may actually, in some cases, have an inflammatory autoimmune component with systemic effects.[6] In addition, researchers estimate up to 78 percent of patients with IBS have underlying SIBO. IBS is one of the biggest gut problems tied to inflammation, with a worldwide prevalence between 9 and 14 percent—that's up to one billion people suffering from the biggest and most reversible gut issue, one that leads to chronic, systemic inflammation.[7]

*Time* magazine once called chronic inflammation "the silent killer," and they weren't exaggerating. Most of the damage done in the body by chronic inflammation begins at the cellular level years before you even realize you have a problem. By the time any disease manifests, inflammation has been running rampant for years or even decades. You don't go from having *no disease* to suddenly having *a disease*.

Rheumatoid arthritis, psoriasis, allergies, asthma, hives, Crohn's disease, and ulcerative colitis are all the result of a chronic inflammatory response.[8] Inflammation is also the leading cause of aging, because chronic inflammatory conditions result in free radicals that damage DNA, which in turn is one of the main drivers of cellular aging.[9] Think of it this way: **When you're aging and inflamed, you're "inflam-aging."**

The drivers of inflammation in the body—like leaky gut and dysbiosis—are the link between being healthy and having a chronic degenerative condition, and between aging well and aging "well beyond your years." *This means that the gut is not only the biggest potential source of inflammation in the body, it is also the gateway for reversing that inflammation.*

Ultimately, gut dysbiosis and leaky gut impact every system in your body. They activate your immune response, the primary driver of inflammation, and send body-wide alert signals that travel to every tissue in your body. *Why is an immune response along your gut lining so impactful?* It's because most of your immune system resides within your gut. In fact, **gut-associated lymphoid tissue** (GALT)—the part of the immune system found in the approximately 20 feet of your gut lining—accounts for almost 70 percent of your entire immune system.[10]

---

‡ What's the difference between IBS and IBD? IBS and IBD can have some similar gastrointestinal symptoms, but IBS is milder and considered a functional bowel disorder, whereas IBD can cause destructive inflammation of the intestinal lining, leading to blood mixed with the stool, incapacitating abdominal pain, more extensive body-wide symptoms, and an increased risk for colon cancer.

When your gut-associated immune system is distracted by a constant onslaught of inflammation-inducing substances coming through a leaky gut barrier, it weakens your defenses against viruses and bacterial infections in other parts of your body, most commonly the respiratory system. This leads to an increased risk of respiratory infections—just like what happened to me when I was a child. To understand this better, let's take a closer look at how leaky gut works.

## LEAKY GUT, EXPLAINED

I want to make sure I don't lose you at this point, because this is one of the most important concepts you need to understand to begin healing not just your gut, but also the rest of your body. When we work on leaky gut syndrome, patients are often surprised at how many other seemingly unrelated symptoms improve.

Let's start with a simple analogy that helps explain how leaky gut works:

*Your gut lining functions much the same way as a coffee filter.* Imagine making a cup of pour-over coffee. As you pour the hot water over the coffee grounds inside the coffee filter, you want the water to pass through the filtered grounds so that you get a pure, beautiful, aromatic cup of coffee-infused water without the coffee grounds. The filter is what makes that possible: It lets the water pass through while keeping the coffee grounds from falling into the mug.

*Now, imagine that the coffee filter is your gut lining, and the food you're eating is the coffee grounds.* Your gut lining (the coffee filter) lets through the nutrients extracted from your food (the coffee-infused water), while keeping all the unnecessary and harmful stuff you don't need (the coffee grounds) inside the **gut lumen**—the opening inside the bowels through which food that is being digested passes and eventually is turned into stool. This is what happens when your gut is working as intended.

*But let's say I take that coffee filter and poke holes in it with a toothpick to simulate a leaky gut.* Now that there are multiple tiny holes in the filter, when you pour the water over it, coffee grounds get through and into your cup. So instead of a delicious cup of aromatic coffee, you have a cup of sludge. That's the whole idea behind leaky gut—things that shouldn't get through the gut lining do get through, bogging up your system with "sludge." And unfortunately, when that happens, a whole slew of health problems tends to follow.

## COFFEE FILTER ANALOGY
### LEAKY GUT vs. HEALTHY GUT

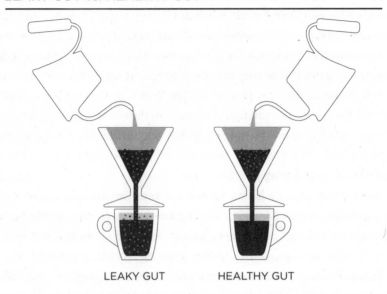

LEAKY GUT          HEALTHY GUT

Now, you may be wondering: Why is this a problem? Doesn't my body just take care of whatever comes through and clean itself out?

I wish it was that simple. As I explained earlier, the things that can get through a leaky gut barrier activate an inflammatory response. There's a direct connection between leaky gut, your immune system, and inflammation. When the wrong things get through your gut lining, they trigger an immune response that leads to inflammation, and this process causes more and more damage, like an avalanche, leading to almost every chronic, degenerative disease on the planet. Unlike many other medical conditions, which have a small handful of characteristic symptoms, leaky gut syndrome has a plethora of them. This means leaky gut is frequently mistaken for many other conditions. In fact, you can think of leaky gut as the great masquerader.

## LEAKY GUT: THE GREAT MASQUERADER

Leaky gut syndrome has only recently become better understood by researchers, and it's often overlooked by Western medicine doctors, despite the growing body of evidence showcasing its prevalence and potential for harm. And I'll admit, even twenty years ago, leaky gut syndrome sounded to me like a sci-fi condition that had no bearing on human health. Boy, was I wrong! Leaky gut is being brought to light as *the underlying driving factor* behind many chronic degenerative diseases.

Unfortunately, because leaky gut syndrome is often also a silent condition, many people don't realize they're struggling with it until they are very sick. By the time people come to my practice in New York City, they are basically at their wits' end, having reached multiple dead ends in their healing journeys. Leaky gut is a prime example of how "it starts with the gut." And unless you know that the symptoms you're struggling with *could* be coming from your gut, you won't know where to start your healing.

Many conditions we blame on other causes are actually rooted in leaky gut. This is because, as I'll explain in the next chapter, the gut is linked to every organ system, and that means symptoms can manifest almost anywhere in the body—skin, brain, lungs, sinuses, mouth, genitals, bladder . . . you name it.

Studies have shown that leaky gut syndrome can put you at risk for a multitude of diseases (or, if you have a disease already, it can exacerbate symptoms).[11] Autoimmune diseases like inflammatory bowel diseases (Crohn's and ulcerative colitis), celiac disease, autoimmune hepatitis, multiple sclerosis, and systemic lupus erythematosus are just a few of those.[12] They all have one thing in common—a leaky gut. We are even coming to understand that a subset of IBS may actually be caused by an autoimmune reaction triggered in the gut by certain types of bacteria. These diseases compromise the quality of life and can even decrease life expectancy by triggering *inflam-aging* (as discussed above).[13]

So, if leaky gut syndrome is the great masquerader, how are you supposed to know if you have it? First, take an inventory of your symptoms.

## THE SYMPTOMS OF LEAKY GUT SYNDROME

The symptoms of leaky gut syndrome can be divided into two large categories: *gut-centric symptoms* (ones that happen inside the gut) and *gut-related symptoms* (ones that happen outside the gut).

## What Is a Gut-Centric Symptom?

Gut-centric symptoms tend to be the more obvious ones that come to mind when we think of digestion. These include **bloating, abdominal pain, diarrhea, cramping, constipation,** and **mucus and/or blood in the stool.** (To be clear, when I say blood in the stool, I mean blood mixed with the stool, not in addition to it, like you might experience with hemorrhoids, which can result in bright red blood in the toilet bowl and on the toilet paper when you wipe.)[‡]

Because **gut-centric symptoms** occur in the gut—as in, they manifest in organs located around the gut—when we experience them, we have a general idea of where they're likely coming from. But it's not always that straightforward.

## Caution: "Gut-centric" symptoms may sometimes be *unrelated* to the gut.

What do I mean by this? Let's use a stomachache as an example.

When you get a stomachache, you physically feel the pain in your stomach region (or at least in your abdomen generally). Naturally, you assume the pain is caused by whatever's going on in your stomach. You wouldn't think for a second that your heart or kidneys were the reason your stomach is hurting because the pain is localized to your abdominal region. Even if you had an underlying heart condition, you'd probably think it was just something you ate. However, some heart attacks can present with a feeling of indigestion in the upper part of the stomach that won't go away, and a passing kidney stone can first show up as acute abdominal pain.

Gut-centric symptoms can also sometimes be related to referred pain from an internal organ or muscle. This happened to a patient of mine, Hayley, who had a history of IBD and went to see her gastroenterologist for abdominal pain that wasn't following her usual pattern. A stool test didn't indicate she was having a flare-up, but since she went to see a GI specialist, he still thought her IBD was the problem. She came to see me for a second opinion, and when I examined her, it became

---

‡ If you experience blood in your stool in any of the ways described here, this is something you should take seriously. Please see a medical doctor for an evaluation, diagnosis, and treatment plan.

apparent there was a muscular component to her complaint. I decided to check if the pain she was feeling would be reproducible through deep palpation of the psoas muscle—a key muscle involved in walking and flexing of the hip joint. The psoas attaches to the hip joint and sends fingerlike attachments all up the lumbar spine, behind the abdominal organs. This muscle can get very tight from extended sitting, and Hayley was a student at the time, taking graduate-level courses. When the tips of my fingers touched her right psoas muscle, she nearly jumped off the table. I'd reproduced the exact abdominal pain she had seen her gastroenterologist about.

Understanding when, how, and where to look for the root cause(s) of symptoms is a key step in discovering whether a person is suffering from leaky gut syndrome. And it's important to also know that not every abdominal symptom may be coming from the gut itself, even though most of them are.

In general, the symptoms you feel within your abdomen are *most likely* related to a gut issue.

The confusion around leaky gut syndrome—what makes it tricky to recognize and difficult to diagnose—has more to do with **gut-related symptoms** . . . especially when those gut-related symptoms show up **in the absence of gut-centric symptoms**. In the next chapter, we tackle some gut-related symptoms and interconnections that may surprise you, but will also show you that starting with the gut as the *cornerstone of your health* is the foundation for healing. Whether you are experiencing a gut-centric symptom or gut-related symptom, the best place to start healing is the gut.

## A WORD OF REASSURANCE

I realize that was probably a lot to take in (and there's more to come)! If you feel overwhelmed at all, please know that what you're feeling is normal, and okay. I struggled with my gut health for over two decades and had to navigate through a long gut-healing journey to get to where I am now. But your journey doesn't have to be as long as mine—that is the focus and goal of this book!

If it turns out you do have leaky gut syndrome, please know that it's much more common than you think, and there's plenty you can do to heal! To be honest, I'm usually a bit relieved when I discover a patient's symptoms are being caused by leaky gut syndrome. They are usually shocked that their gut is the source of their problems (especially if they don't have any gut-centric symptoms), and sometimes they're frustrated that it took so long to pinpoint the underlying issue—but having a diagnosis and plan of action gives them a sense of relief and reassurance.

So whether this is the first or millionth thing you've tried, you can feel good knowing that this book is here to help you. If you have ever felt like giving up on improving your health, let me be the person who tells you not to. I hope the fact that I'm here writing this for you serves as assurance that you *can get better* and that even long-standing symptoms can be resolved and are not a reason to throw in the towel just yet.

The recommendations I make in this book are the same I would (and do) give to my patients, family, friends, and myself. They're backed by decades of research and patient care. I wrote this book so you could feel like you are finally in good hands, and if you can stay positive and focused, you're already halfway there.

## Takeaways

At the end of each chapter, I'll give you a few major highlights that you should take with you as you continue reading this book. Think of these as the "if you learned anything from this chapter" sticking points.

1. The GutSMART Protocol is a 14-day actionable food-based gut-healing plan that is individualized according to the results of the GutSMART Quiz.

2. The gut is where you have to begin when it comes to healing your body, starting from the inside out.

3. Dysbiosis is an imbalance between favorable and unfavorable microorganisms in the gut, where the scale is tipped toward the unfavorable ones.

4. There are multiple potential types of dysbiosis: an excess of bad bacteria, of yeast, of parasites, or of worms, or any combination of these.

5. For the purposes of this book, when I say "dysbiosis," I am referring to an overgrowth of bad bacteria in the gut, which may or may not be accompanied by a yeast imbalance or parasites.

6. Your gut lining functions much the same way as a coffee filter. Increased intestinal permeability, or **leaky gut**, is an impairment of the semipermeable intestinal barrier that, like a coffee filter with holes poked in it, lets more through than it should.

7. The causes of leaky gut include antibiotics, autoimmune disease, birth control pills, common OTC medications (like NSAID painkillers and antacids), dysbiosis, gastrointestinal infections, low stomach acid, pesticides, poor diet (high in processed foods), stress, and toxins.

8. When your gut becomes "leaky," the connections between the cells that line your intestinal wall and help keep the barrier sealed (known as **tight junctions**) become looser, allowing larger molecules—like partially digested food proteins, bacteria, bacterial DNA, yeast, and even parasites—to pass through.

9. The symptoms of leaky gut syndrome can be divided into two large categories: *gut-centric symptoms* (ones that happen inside the gut) and *gut-related symptoms* (ones that happen outside the gut).

10. Leaky gut causes inflammation, and chronic inflammation puts you at risk for countless diseases and conditions, especially autoimmune diseases.

11. Inflammation is at the root of every disease in the body. And the gut is your biggest potential source of inflammation.

Chapter 2

# FIX YOUR GUT, FIX YOUR BODY

## The 7 Categories of Leaky Gut Symptoms

> *"Unlike in Vegas, what happens in the gut doesn't stay in the gut."*
>
> —*Dr. Vincent Pedre*

**While the gut-centric symptoms of leaky gut occur inside the gut** (and so are easier to spot), **gut-related symptoms** occur **outside of the gut**—meaning that, while they happen elsewhere in the body, the underlying issue that's causing them resides in the gut. In other words, problems in the gut don't stay in the gut; they can have major effects on the rest of your body, and even your metabolism and immune system.

I personally divide these leaky-gut related symptoms into seven different categories based on where they show up or what aspect of the body they affect:

- Skin
- Airway

- Brain
- Joints
- Energy
- Metabolism
- Immune system

Let's look at each of these in turn, starting with the skin—one of the most well-researched of these gut-connected categories.

## THE GUT-SKIN CONNECTION

If you're dealing with skin issues, there's a good chance you've already seen your primary care doctor and a dermatologist (maybe even more than one). You may feel like you've exhausted all your options. I see patients all the time who feel like their skin condition is a life sentence and there's nothing they can do about it except take a daily antibiotic, use topical remedies, or try birth control pills.

But here's something a conventional doctor won't tell you:

. . . . . . . . . . . . . . . . . . . . . . . . . . . . . . . . . . . . . . . . . . . . . . . . . . . . .

### The way your body looks on the *outside* is a direct reflection of what's happening on the *inside*.

. . . . . . . . . . . . . . . . . . . . . . . . . . . . . . . . . . . . . . . . . . . . . . . . . . . . .

And in the case of skin conditions, what's happening on the inside is almost always an undiagnosed gut health issue that is showing up as inflammation, redness, flaking, or an allergic reaction. That's why I like to call the gut our *inner skin*. There is an intimate, bidirectional connection between the gut and skin that influences the skin's optimal functioning and modulates the skin's immune response to the outside world.[1] Leaky gut syndrome can show up on your skin in the form of **acne, rashes, hives, eczema, seborrheic dermatitis**, and **psoriasis**, thanks to the increase in inflammation it causes in the body.[2] Leaky gut also leads to hormone imbalances and can even contribute to psychological stress, both of which lead to—you guessed it!—the worsening of any skin condition.[3]

Also, believe it or not, the skin barrier itself actually becomes "leaky" in some of these conditions, including eczema and psoriasis. When the skin barrier is functioning properly, it has the ability to limit evaporation, preserve skin moisture, and protect us from invasion by foreign organisms and substances like bacteria.[4] The skin is able to do this, however, only when the rest of the body is in **homeostasis** (a word that refers to a positive equilibrium between interdependent elements—in effect, the opposite of dysbiosis). *And can you guess what plays a large role in that homeostasis?* The gut! Studies have shown that when the intestinal barrier is disturbed (as in leaky gut), intestinal bacteria and their metabolites gain access to the bloodstream. From there, they can accumulate in the skin and disrupt skin homeostasis.[5]

If you're like most of my patients, this is news to you—and it may sound kind of out there. But let me assure you that this connection is well established. The last two decades of scientific research have connected alterations in the gut microbiome to a myriad of skin conditions, including: acne vulgaris,[6] rosacea,[7] atopic dermatitis, and psoriasis.[8] The authors of one study[9] even explain that the gut microbiota communicate directly with the skin. This is especially true for **acne**.

## Acne & Your Gut

Nisha came in to see me because of unrelenting cystic adult acne on her face and upper back. After visiting multiple dermatologists, she was frustrated that the topical remedies weren't working. During her visit, we talked about the gut-skin connection and addressed dietary factors that might be playing a role. Through an elimination diet, we discovered that dairy was a major culprit. By removing dairy products from her diet (not an easy feat, since she loved to eat cheese and protein bars that had dairy in them), her acne improved within weeks. She also noticed that her bowel movements became more regular. Of course, we also had to work on healing the gut lining and lowering her stress levels (another big trigger for acne), but we made a huge leap forward by finding her food trigger. And her better skin health offered a huge confidence boost.

If you've been battling with adult acne and have spent a lot of time and money trying to fix the problem from the outside with topical remedies, you might have been told that acne is caused by "bad bacteria" on the skin. Acne has been connected to skin dysbiosis with the *Cutibacterium acnes* species of bacteria and an increase in other types of bacteria.[10] But as the authors of a study published in

2020 explain: "The interactions between the bacteria involved in acne extend beyond the skin itself."[11]

. . . . . . . . . . . . . . . . . . . . . . . . . . . . . . . . . . . . . . . . . . . . .

## Research has shown that patients with acne have different concentrations of certain gut bacteria than patients without acne, which make them more prone to skin inflammation.

. . . . . . . . . . . . . . . . . . . . . . . . . . . . . . . . . . . . . . . . . . . . .

Therefore, the true underlying cause of acne lies both locally on the skin and distantly in the gut, since the balance of good and bad bacteria in the gut microbiome plays a significant role in skin health. Moreover, scientists have even been able to connect acne to specific strains of gut bacteria. For example, a study of thirty-one acne patients showed that the bacterial strain *Actinobacteria* was less abundant and *Proteobacteria* was more abundant in the guts of people with acne.[12]

So what causes these imbalances? Acne's proximate causes include hormone imbalances, diet, and stress—all factors that are closely connected to the gut.

**Hormone imbalances:** Underlying hormone imbalances, like *estrogen dominance* or *polycystic ovarian syndrome* (PCOS), have been shown to contribute to acne, and frequently go undiagnosed. Your gut can either promote hormone balance or aggravate hormone imbalances. One way the gut does this is through a group of bacteria collectively known as the *estrobolome*. As the name implies, they help metabolize estrogens (both those produced by the body and estrogen-like compounds, otherwise known as *xenobiotics* or EDCs—*endocrine-disrupting chemicals*—from the environment) in order to support hormone balance, especially for women. Sometimes a dysbiosis leads to an overgrowth of certain bacteria that produce an enzyme that frees up metabolized estrogen in the stool to recirculate back into the body, causing estrogen dominance and leading to acne.

**Diet:** Certain foods have been linked to an increased incidence of acne. For example, a meta-analysis of fourteen different studies showed a significant link between dairy products (including milk chocolate) and an increased likelihood of acne. In addition, high-sugar foods that increase the secretion of *insulin* (your blood sugar–balancing hormone)—simple carbs like candy, bread, pastries, cakes, and pasta—contribute to acne as well by causing a dysbiosis that leads to a leaky gut.

**Stress:** Emotional stress has been connected to increases in both acne incidence and severity. Stress is like an attack on your gut. It increases the likelihood of leaky gut, and high stress will even shift your gut flora to more unfavorable bacteria that can trigger acne. Often, you may be doing everything right with diet and supplements, but if you're not addressing stress, you're missing one key component to gut healing that will affect your skin (and so much more). (We'll cover stress and your gut in more detail in Part IV.)

All of these factors can contribute to the development and severity of acne individually; and collectively, they have one thing in common—they're all connected to the gut. *Heal your gut, and your acne will follow.*

## Rosacea & Your Gut

While acne is one of the biggest skin conditions worldwide, affecting 9.4 percent of the world population (over 750 million people!),[13] it's far from the only skin issue heavily impacted by gut health. Rosacea is another example.

**Rosacea** is a common skin condition, affecting 5.46 percent of the world population (approximately 436 million people).[14] It typically manifests as redness in the center of the face, especially around the nose and anterior cheeks, but it can also affect the forehead and chin, and is characterized by visible blood vessels and small, red bumps that can be mistaken for acne, swelling of the tissue of the nose (making the nose look bigger), and swelling and redness around the eyelids. From the functional medicine point of view, rosacea is caused by excess inflammation and a dysregulation of the immune system—both of which are directly connected to the gut.

If you go to a conventional doctor for rosacea, they will tell you that there's no cure and that the best thing they can do is help you control symptoms during a flare-up. They will prescribe a topical antibiotic (like metronidazole gel) that can reduce redness of the skin and blood vessels, or oral medications such as antibiotics or isotretinoin (which are also used for acne) to reduce skin dysbiosis and inflammation, helping to modulate the skin's immune response. But these conventional treatments for rosacea neglect to address the true underlying cause—and can have unpleasant secondary consequences, like they did for my patient John.

John had been prescribed a topical antibiotic for rosacea by another doctor and came to see me complaining of gut problems—gas, bloating, and loose stools. He appeared to have developed "IBS" as a side effect of the topical antibiotic (not a known side effect of this treatment, but not outside the realm of possibility). So instead of treating his rosacea topically, we took him off the topical remedy and started him on a gut-healing regimen. This included modifying his diet to remove food triggers, while introducing other foods to improve the health of his gut lining and the diversity of his gut microbiome. Not only did his rosacea improve, but his gut health did too. He hadn't realized how bad his gut had been until his digestion felt better than ever.

## Other Skin Conditions & Your Gut

**Psoriasis** is a chronic, immune-mediated, inflammatory skin condition. Patients with psoriasis have been shown to have a depletion of symbiotic gut microbes in comparison to non-psoriatic patients, suggesting that gut dysbiosis may lead and/or contribute to psoriasis's development.[15] Similar to psoriasis, in the case of **eczema** (another inflammatory skin condition, also called *atopic dermatitis*), studies have shown that the primary players in its development are skin barrier dysfunction and altered immune responses.[16] And by now you know what causes skin barrier dysfunction and immune activation: leaky gut!

That was the case for my patient Juan. He came in with severe eczema around his mouth, eyes, and knuckles. No doctor had been able to find the underlying root cause, and he was tired of treating it with topical remedies that worked when he used them but then allowed the eczema to keep coming back whenever he stopped. It turned out he was allergic to wheat, dairy, corn, and soy. In addition, he had an intestinal dysbiosis and was infected with parasites. By removing the food triggers in his diet and treating the underlying root cause of his inflammatory skin condition—the parasites and leaky gut stemming from the dysbiosis—his skin improved within one month, and by following the GutSMART Protocol you'll learn in Part II, Juan was able to maintain healthy skin thereafter.

# THE GUT-AIRWAY CONNECTION

The gut-related symptoms you might see in your nasal passages, sinuses, trachea, and lungs include **postnasal drip, sinus congestion, dry cough, asthma, allergies,** and **susceptibility to sinus and lung infections** (see "The Gut-Immune Connection" on page 49 for more).

A 2020 review of multiple studies underscored the influence of the gut microbiome on the respiratory system.[17] Several of the studies involved older people (mostly in their sixties and seventies), because aging is associated with dysbiosis and loss of resilience and diversity of the gut microbiota. The elderly are also especially susceptible to lung diseases and infections. The researchers found that gut health has a direct impact on the lungs and overall respiratory health, and noted that probiotic bacteria are key players in the maintenance of healthy lungs.

There was also a study in 2020 that showed a correlation between the gut microbiome and the SARS-CoV-2 virus (aka COVID-19), which normally presents with many respiratory symptoms—cough, shortness of breath, difficulty breathing, loss of smell, and congestion or runny nose.[18] This correlation isn't all that surprising when you consider that while many symptoms associated with COVID-19 are respiratory, other observed symptoms involve the digestive system, like nausea and diarrhea. In fact, I had multiple patients who presented with accompanying gut symptoms when they contracted COVID-19. Researchers in the study found that the gut microbiota composition of a patient with COVID-19, even after disease resolution, could determine the severity of their symptoms. Lack of inflammation-fighting gut bacteria in these patients resulted in a higher risk of severe infection and hospitalization. Not a coincidence!

# THE GUT-BRAIN CONNECTION

When Cynthia came to see me for her migraines, I knew we had to investigate what was going on in her gut. While she had done *elimination diets* before (diets that remove the most common food allergens, sensitivities, and intolerances), her migraines persisted. So, I did food sensitivity testing, and to our surprise, out of all the foods, spices, and condiments she could have been sensitive to, she was highly sensitive to cinnamon. Well, she was putting cinnamon on the oatmeal she ate almost every day. By removing cinnamon from her diet (while also working on a broader gut-healing protocol), her migraine frequency immediately dropped by 50 percent in the first month. This was a huge relief to Cynthia, and just one example of the power of the gut-brain connection.

In a 2016 study, researchers in Turkey found that certain foods were migraine-triggering for different patients.[19] Once those foods were determined for each patient, the patient eliminated them from their diets for several months. After the first month alone, the frequency, duration, and severity of their migraines all decreased, a result that was sustained for the remainder of the study in the group that continued to strictly eliminate migraine-triggering foods. Subsequent studies have confirmed these findings, and it's now generally accepted that headaches and migraines are responsive to diet and can be triggered by the gut's reaction to certain foods.[20]

It's also well documented that many gastrointestinal disorders can cause frequent headaches and migraines.[21] Among those disorders are irritable bowel syndrome (IBS), celiac disease, and constipation.

The relationship between the gut and the brain is often referred to as the **gut-brain axis** or **gut-brain connection** and is one of the most powerful relationships in the body. It begins when we are in utero, and it influences our brain health both in the short term (like our productivity and ability to focus) and in the long term (like our memory and cognitive function as we age). It also plays a significant role in our mental health.

## Mental Health & Your Gut

The gut-brain connection has a major, yet underappreciated, influence on our mental state. In the last five years alone, numerous prominent studies have demonstrated the link between gut health and the prevention and treatment of mental illnesses.[22] Research in this area is becoming more robust every single day, showing not only that the diversity and abundance of gut bacteria affect overall health but that there is direct, bidirectional communication between the brain and the gut that impacts how our brain functions and how we feel, as well as how the gut functions (more on this relationship in chapter 10). According to a paper published in 2017, dysregulation in the gut-brain axis—like what occurs when you develop a leaky gut—can lead to mental health and sensory processing disorders. "For instance, altered microbiota has been linked to neuropsycholog-ical disorders including depression and autism spectrum disorder," the authors wrote.[23]

If you've ever struggled with a mental health issue—whether it is anxiety, depression, OCD, panic attacks, or any other condition—I want you to know first that I see you, and I understand how tough it is to struggle with mental health. I've had my own tough mental challenges that, looking back, were related to my poor gut health. When you're in the thick of it, it can feel lonely and really hard. Know that you are not alone.

Mental illness is incredibly common, affecting up to 50 million Americans and anywhere between 11 and 18 percent of people globally (that's up to a whopping 1.4 billion people!),[24] yet therapies that *really* work are severely lacking. That's where focusing on gut microbiota for therapeutic purposes comes into play, in an emerg-ing field of probiotic therapy known as psychobiotics. **Psychobiotics** are friendly gut bacteria that have been found to offer mental health benefits when taken orally.

For example, one study showed that administration of the probiotic *Lactoba-cillus rhamnosus* to mice resulted in reduced anxiety- and depressive-like behaviors and led to long-term positive changes, allowing for a more balanced functioning of the central nervous system.[25] In another study, women volunteered to drink a fermented milk product (like kefir) rich in probiotic bacteria for a four-week period while tracking their brains' responses via functional magnetic resonance imaging (fMRI) before and after the four weeks.[26] The results showed that the probiotic-rich drink influenced brain activity in the emotional centers, something that can in turn lower anxiety.[27]

Another study showed that consuming *Bifidobacterium longum* for four weeks reduced production of the stress hormone **cortisol** in response to stressors, in addition to reducing subjective anxiety and daily stress.[28] Finally, multiple stud-ies[29] have shown that certain bacteria can help reverse depression.

The gut has a **circular relationship** with various mental health conditions, including chronic stress, depression, and anxiety,[30] as well as psychiatric disor-ders, like bipolar disorder, schizophrenia, and autism spectrum disorder.[31] What I mean by *circular relationship* is that an unbalanced gut flora or poor gut health can contribute to mental illness, but mental illness can also cause the gut to become unbalanced and gut health to worsen. Contrary to its name, mental illness isn't confined to the brain. As you know if you've ever experienced stress, anxiety, or depression, the physical symptoms of mental illness are very real, and those symptoms often take place in the gut—think upset stomach, abdominal pain, diarrhea, constipation, bloating, IBS, etc.

Bottom line: The brain can affect the structure and health of the gut (including the gut lining via the vagus nerve—stuff we'll get into later when I talk about ways you can turbocharge your results in chapter 10), and the gut can affect brain function as well. That's why we say that their relationship is circular or bidirectional: It goes both ways.[32]

## The Aging Brain & Your Gut

This gut-brain connection plays an important role in the development and prevention of neurological diseases and disorders.[33] In particular, studies have shown that gut microbiota have a direct effect on central nervous system disorders like autism spectrum disorder,[34] learning disabilities, and mood disorders (like depression and anxiety).[35] Similarly, poor gut health has been linked to the development of neurodegenerative disorders that develop later in life—like **Alzheimer's** and **dementia**.[36]

An estimated 5.8 million Americans ages sixty-five and over currently suffer from Alzheimer's disease—and the Centers for Disease Control (CDC) predicts that number will triple by 2060, to nearly 14 million. According to the World Health Organization, currently 55 million people worldwide are living with dementia, and there are 10 million new cases of it every year.[37] For decades, we thought Alzheimer's was solely a genetic condition and that there was no way to prevent it—and no treatment or cure. Thankfully, the latest research suggests that our gut health can affect our risk of developing diseases like Alzheimer's to begin with, as well as their severity once developed.

Speaking of the latest research, a recent study from researchers at the University of Lund in Sweden found that mice suffering from an Alzheimer's-like condition had a different composition of gut bacteria compared to healthy mice.[38] Why is this significant? Well, the researchers saw that mice with no gut bacteria (aka "germ-free" mice) had significantly fewer **beta-amyloid plaques** (lumps that form around Alzheimer's patients' brain nerve fibers) in their brains than the mice with Alzheimer's. When the researchers transferred bacteria from the Alzheimer's mice to the germ-free mice, they developed more beta-amyloid plaques than if they had received bacteria from healthy mice. In short, this study suggested that gut bacteria are directly linked to the development of Alzheimer's disease and reaffirmed that the gut-brain connection is worthy of our attention when it comes to the aging brain.

## Your Brain and Leaky Gut

If you ever wondered where that **brain fog** is coming from, it's most likely your gut. As we've already discussed, other common leaky gut symptoms affecting the head and brain include **headaches**, **migraines**, and mental health issues like **depression** and **anxiety**. Remember: Leaky gut never happens on its own; it's usually accompanied by a dysbiosis. While not every dysbiosis involves yeast overgrowth, many do, and the mycotoxins produced by this overgrowth can often lead you to feel like you're in a foggy cloud all day, struggling to focus and get through your workday.

Two big issues that are important to mention here, because they can also result in headaches, migraines, and brain fog, are food sensitivities and intolerances. Food sensitivities are connected to our stomach acid and enzyme production. Stomach acid is what helps break down the proteins in our food into amino acids that the body needs as the building blocks of tissues, muscle, and neurotransmitters. When the body is unable to do that because of inadequate stomach acid and digestive enzymes, our food isn't broken down properly. Combine that with leaky gut, and partially digested proteins get through the gut lining, thus triggering an immune response. The result? A food sensitivity or allergy, symptoms of which may include headaches, migraines, fatigue, joint aches, and/or brain fog.

As I'm sure you're starting to understand, things in the body don't happen in isolation. I first started noticing this almost two decades ago when I took note that pretty much every migraine patient also complained of IBS-like symptoms. I paid special attention to patterns (something I'm going to ask of you later) and started making the connection between the two conditions. So, whereas we can talk about the specific interconnections between the gut and brain separately from other systems, every system, symptom, and disease in the body is in reality interconnected, and I hope this book is helping you appreciate that better.

### Food Intolerance, Food Sensitivity, or Food Allergy?

People get the terms *food intolerance*, *food sensitivity*, and *food allergy* confused a lot—it's one of the most common questions I get from my patients. So, I wanted to take a second to clear up the differences.

**Food intolerance** describes an inability to properly digest a certain food. The most common example worldwide is lactose intolerance, which affects up to 90 percent of people of Asian, African, Hispanic, or Native American descent. When you are *lactose intolerant*, it means the cells that form the inner lining of the small intestine don't produce enough of the lactase enzyme needed to break down the lactose found in dairy products. The result is gas and bloating. You can also have a *fructose intolerance* (a problem absorbing fruit sugar) and even a wheat intolerance. That's where it gets a little confusing—because you can also have a *wheat sensitivity*.

When you develop a **food sensitivity**, it means your body produces a specific type of immune response to that food, called an IgG response. This type of response is slow and may not show up for hours or even days after eating the food. IgGs are antibodies that are found *only* in your bloodstream. So, the only way for you to develop a food sensitivity is to develop a leaky gut first. The pathway to food sensitivities *always* involves leaky gut, because leaky gut is what allows partially digested food proteins to enter your bloodstream and activate your immune response.

In contrast to a sensitivity, a *wheat intolerance* is due to an issue with the *fructans* (short-chain sugars) in wheat that, instead of getting broken down by our enzymes, get fermented by gut bacteria, resulting in uncomfortable gas, bloating, and even diarrhea. (**Wheat intolerance** is just one of many FODMAP issues—problems digesting certain types of dietary sugars known as Fermentable Oligo-, Di-, Monosaccharides, And Polyols.) Wheat intolerance doesn't have to cause an immune reaction, as in a sensitivity, but it can still lead to GI distress. There are a lot of foods you can be intolerant to because of a FODMAP issue, but that doesn't necessarily mean that you are sensitive to that food. And vice versa! You may be sensitive to a food but not have an intolerance to it. Or you might have both.

A **food allergy**, like a food sensitivity, happens when your body develops an immune response to a food. What makes it different from a sensitivity are three things:

1. *the type of immune response*—Food allergies are mediated by IgE, not IgG, antibodies.

2. *the rapidity of the response*—It can be immediate: within seconds to minutes.

3. *the relationship to leaky gut*—Food allergies do not require a leaky gut to develop.

Often, food allergies are inherited, whereas food sensitivities can be acquired—though some food allergies can be acquired as well. It can get confusing, but remember the basics above.

Is leaky gut involved with food intolerances? It's complicated. You don't need to have a leaky gut to develop a food intolerance. It's just based on your ability to break down certain nutrients—which may actually depend on the makeup of your gut flora. An intolerance usually happens because you don't make enough enzymes in your gut to break down the food, and that inability can be inherited. But it can also be acquired—the result of a dysbiosis in your gut microbiome. If you do have a leaky gut, that could be what's causing the enzyme deficiency (leading to the food intolerance, and eventually, potentially a sensitivity to that food).

See why it's so crucial to heal your gut? I wasn't kidding—it impacts *everything*!

# THE GUT-JOINT CONNECTION

Swati came to see me feeling distraught after being diagnosed with an undefined autoimmune condition, characterized by a whole host of problems: high autoimmune antibodies, joint aches, hives, and chronic fatigue. She had a four-year-old son, and she thought at first that the fatigue and achiness were related to being a mom. However, in the year since she'd moved to the US from India, she had developed a complicated array of symptoms that seemed to have no unifying explanation, particularly the migrating joint pain and hives.

Numerous studies have demonstrated a link between the composition of gut microbes and joint-related diseases and conditions, including *rheumatoid arthritis*,[39] which causes swelling, pain, stiffness, and loss of function in joints; and *osteoarthritis*, which can result in joint degeneration, inflammation, pain, and disability.[40] Once again, this is an example of how dysbiosis and leaky gut are associated with the development of inflammatory diseases, and why I suspected that Swati's symptoms, although not in the gut, were related to her gut health.[41]

Surprisingly, Swati *didn't* complain of any gut-centric symptoms at all.

You can imagine the extensive work-up Swati had done before her diagnosis, including ruling out Lyme disease. Doctors wanted to put her on strong immunosuppressives and monoclonal antibodies to treat her symptoms. However, she instinctively knew that wasn't the long-term answer for her problems, and even though she lacked any gut symptoms, she looked toward her gut as the key to the solution.

One month before meeting with me for the first time, she read my book *Happy Gut* and began the suggested elimination diet, cutting out both dairy and wheat. By the time she saw me for her first appointment, the hives had diminished by 75 percent, but she was still experiencing joint pain and fatigue. I diagnosed her with leaky gut syndrome and a dysbiosis with parasites and yeast overgrowth. By treating these underlying conditions, her joint pain completely disappeared and her energy returned to pre-pregnancy levels. The *most important takeaway* from Swati's story is that you shouldn't be fooled if you don't have gut symptoms; joint aches and pains could still be related to your gut and leaky gut syndrome.

# THE GUT-ENERGY CONNECTION

"I have no energy!" is a complaint I have heard hundreds of times in my twenty years of doctoring. Fatigue is something that affects your whole body, instead of feeling it in specific organs or body parts—you feel it everywhere. Symptoms can range from **low energy** and **muscle aches** to the **post-meal food coma** (discussed below). And while lack of energy is usually associated with low thyroid function, unaddressed gut issues are often a major contributing factor, because the gut is the root system of the body, and the effective absorption of micronutrients is a must-have for optimal energy.

One key problem that arises when you have a leaky gut is that the nutrients from the foods you eat don't get broken down and absorbed properly. I know it may not make sense that when the gut is leakier, micronutrients can't get through as easily, but that is exactly the case.[42, 43, 44] When we eat, the acid in our stomach works in combination with the digestive enzymes produced by the stomach, pancreas, and inner lining of the small intestine, as well as the trillions of microbes in the large intestine, to break down food and extract its nutrients. The fats, carbs, and proteins in food can't be absorbed and utilized by the body until they're broken down into their component parts. Without a healthy gut, digestion and absorption plummet. When you're not properly digesting or absorbing the nutrients to produce all the energy your body needs, you feel—as I did for years—tired and unmotivated.

Gut health also impacts how metabolic byproducts and toxins are eliminated from the body, which affects our energy levels as well.[45] When the gut becomes leaky—when the gut lining because more permeable—toxins and inflammatory molecules gain entry into the body, where they can cause significant damage. **Mitochondria**, the hundreds (sometimes thousands) of energy factories inside every cell in your body, are particularly sensitive to damage from these toxins. And when mitochondria stop functioning properly, your energy takes a nosedive.

(I'll go into more detail about the role the gut microbiome plays in energy production in the next chapter.)

# THE GUT-METABOLISM CONNECTION

Our **metabolism** comprises all the life-sustaining chemical reactions that help our bodies run efficiently. We associate a *slow metabolism* with weight gain, and in that context, we tend to think of our metabolism as something that can be affected by only a few factors: our weight, our muscle mass, our hormones, what we eat, how much we exercise, and our genetics. While these aspects certainly do impact metabolism, the health of our gut plays a more vital role than we previously realized. It's often the one missing link for people who are striving to achieve a healthy weight. And the common thread that ties together gut health and weight gain is a tiny molecule you may have never heard of before called **lipopolysaccharide** (LPS), otherwise known as *endotoxin*.[46]

Ever feel a wave of mental fog, like you can barely keep your eyes open, after a meal? We call it a *post-meal food coma*, and it's something I run into a lot with my patients. It results from **diet-induced endotoxemia**—a tidal wave of immune activation and inflammation usually occurring within 30 to 60 minutes after you eat, while your gut is digesting and absorbing nutrients. Its cause? *Endotoxin* escaping the gut and getting absorbed by the body.

**Endotoxin** is a toxin present in the cell membrane of certain bacteria in the gut (typically gram-negative ones, like the infamous *E. coli*) that protects the bacteria from attack and helps reinforce the structural integrity of their membranes. It was originally believed to be released only when these bacteria died, but it was later discovered that living bacteria secrete endotoxin into their surrounding environment as well. Endotoxins are prevalent in the environment—in dust, animal waste, foods, and other materials derived from bacterial products or exposed to them—and for that reason can be inadvertently ingested and found in the gastrointestinal tract. So most of our endotoxin exposure comes from our own gut bacteria.[47] Once in our gut, endotoxins can be absorbed by our gut lining and enter the bloodstream, where they activate the immune system, initiating an inflammatory response within multiple organs, including the brain.

Diet-induced endotoxemia is fueled by diets that are high in sugar, flour, refined carbs, and unhealthy omega-6 vegetable oils,[48] because these foods either feed endotoxin-releasing bacteria or provide a fatty carrier to bring endotoxin into the body. People who have moderate or severe gut dysfunction (see chapter 6) are particularly susceptible to diet-induced endotoxemia because they most certainly

## DIET-INDUCED ENDOTOXEMIA

Endotoxin is a molecule, also known as lipopolysaccharide (LPS), released by certain bacteria in the gut that increases inflammation, insulin resistance, and liver fat, leading to obesity and type 2 diabetes. Eating an inflammatory diet increases endotoxin levels in the blood.

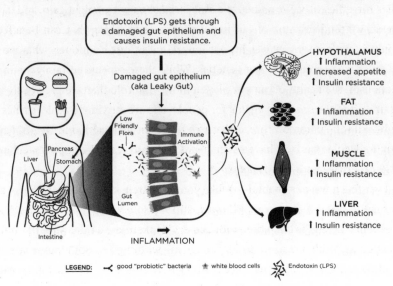

Endotoxin (LPS) gets through a damaged gut epithelium and causes insulin resistance.

Damaged gut epithelium (aka Leaky Gut)

Low Friendly Flora

Immune Activation

Gut Lumen

INFLAMMATION

Pancreas
Liver
Stomach
Intestine

**HYPOTHALAMUS**
↑ Inflammation
↑ Increased appetite
↑ Insulin resistance

**FAT**
↑ Inflammation
↑ Insulin resistance

**MUSCLE**
↑ Inflammation
↑ Insulin resistance

**LIVER**
↑ Inflammation
↑ Insulin resistance

LEGEND: ⤙ good "probiotic" bacteria   ✸ white blood cells   ✵ Endotoxin (LPS)

have leaky gut, and leaky gut makes it easier for these endotoxins to pass through the gut lining.

Why should you care, besides not wanting to feel sleepy after meals? **Studies have shown that a high level of endotoxin in the blood is a precursor for immune-related inflammation, weight gain, obesity, and metabolic syndrome.**[49] Diet-induced endotoxemia is also associated with an increased risk for developing type 2 diabetes,[50] which magnifies the likelihood of heart attacks and stroke.

## THE GUT-IMMUNE CONNECTION

During my teenage years, I suffered from a weak immune system that increased my susceptibility to infections. It was one of the main reasons I wanted to become a doctor—so I could figure out how to not get sick and help others do the same. And when I look back now, I can see the relationship between my constant battle against airway infections like **bronchitis, pneumonia, sinusitis,** and **pharyngitis** and the leaky gut and dysbiosis I was dealing with thanks to my overexposure to antibiotics. (See my full story under *Dr. Pedre's Gut-Healing Journey*.)

Remember, 70 percent of your immune system is found along your gut lining; this is your immune system's "command center." When leaky gut persists for too long, your immune response goes haywire. As unwanted particles—including bacteria, viruses, toxins, undigested food particles, and other substances—enter the bloodstream through the loosened tight junctions in the gut lining, your immune system leaps into action. The effort to fight off these threats activates inflammation in the body.

Your immune system can only fight so many battles before getting overwhelmed. When the immune command center in your gut is constantly bombarded by inflammation-causing substances, it loses its ability to carefully survey and ward off infections in other parts of your body. In essence, the immune system turns on, but is not capable of turning off, leading to further damage and recurrent infections.

If this inflammation becomes chronic, your overstressed immune system begins to misfire. It stops being able to recognize what is self and what isn't self, and starts to attack your own proteins and tissues. Suddenly you're dealing with an **autoimmune disease like Hashimoto's, celiac disease, or rheumatoid arthritis**.

Once I learned about the relationship between the gut and the immune system, I was afraid my gut dysfunction would eventually lead to autoimmune disease, like it did for my mom, who passed away from rheumatoid arthritis, and my older sister, who has multiple sclerosis. It became one of the main motivations to heal my gut.

## LEAKY GUT: HARD TO RECOGNIZE, HARD TO DIAGNOSE

As you can see, leaky gut is complicated! And that can make it hard to recognize, and hard to diagnose.

Even gut-centric symptoms of leaky gut syndrome are often mistakenly attributed to a single issue. For example, if you eat a bowl of dairy-based ice cream and experience bloating and diarrhea, you might assume you're lactose intolerant. But you might instead (or *also*!) be sensitive to dairy proteins (more on that in chapter 7), thanks to background leaky gut.

On the flip side, it's common for people to just ignore the gut-centric symptoms of leaky gut. This becomes harder to do when the symptoms are painful and chronic, but you would be shocked at how many patients I see who have experienced bloating or constipation for decades and just tolerated it or accepted it as their "normal."

I've also had numerous patients come to me, hat in hand, because they've spent years trying to treat symptoms instead of investigating the root cause. Their acne hasn't cleared up with topical remedies or oral antibiotics because the bacteria on their skin is **not** the issue. They can't lose weight no matter how few calories they eat because their caloric intake is **not** the issue.

*Since you picked up this book, I imagine there are some symptoms that you're tired of putting up with, but everything you've tried thus far has let you down.* The good news is that you've come to the right place. Once you determine the degree of your gut-related dysfunction (via the GutSMART Quiz), I'll give you a plan to confront your symptoms head on. Whether you already have a bad case of leaky gut, your gut is just unbalanced and unhappy, or you're riddled with gut-related symptoms, the advice in this book will set you on a path to healing *your gut and body in tandem.*

As this chapter has shown, starting your healing journey with the gut can *not only* beat the bloat and put an end to an "irritated stomach," *but also* resolve many skin issues, balance your hormones, reduce allergies and asthma, improve mental clarity, uplift your mood, boost energy, and even reverse or slow down the progression of chronic diseases, including dementia. (See what I mean? When you start thinking of the gut as the center of the body and you look at the research that's been done, you can see how connected it is to everything.) So many of these symptoms and conditions are a byproduct of not just leaky gut, but also an imbalanced gut microbiome, as I'll dive into in the next chapter.

## Takeaways

Because numerous symptoms throughout the body can be traced back to the gut, that's where we're going to start your healing journey. Keep reading, and we'll get to the bottom of them together.

1. While the gut-centric symptoms of leaky gut occur inside the gut (and so are easier to spot), **gut-related symptoms** occur **outside of the gut**—meaning that, while they happen elsewhere in the body, the underlying issue that's causing them resides in the gut.

2. Leaky gut can cause issues for your skin, airway and respiratory system, brain and mental health, joints, energy, metabolism, and immune system—really, your whole body.

3. The relationship between the gut and the brain—known as the **gut-brain axis** or **gut-brain connection**—is one of the most powerful in the body. It reveals how the gut plays a significant role in our brain and mental health.

4. You don't have to exhibit gut-centric symptoms to have underlying gut imbalances that are manifesting as a systemic inflammatory disorder, including joint pain and autoimmune disease.

5. Your gut controls how you absorb nutrients, which has a trickle-down effect on your energy levels. A leaky gut can lead to poor nutrient absorption, which then causes low energy, muscle aches, and even that post-meal food coma.

6. Leaky gut exposes the body to an inflammatory molecule called endotoxin. High levels of endotoxins in the blood are a precursor for inflammation, weight gain, obesity, and metabolic syndrome.

7. Seventy percent of our immune system is found along our gut lining, making the gut the single biggest potential source of inflammation for the body, affecting every system.

8. Long-standing gut imbalances weaken your defenses against infections.

# Chapter 3

## THE MICROBIOME REVOLUTION

> *"The microbiome affects our mood, libido, metabolism, immunity, and even our perception of the world and the clarity of our thoughts. It helps determine whether we are fat or thin, energic or lethargic. Put simply, everything about our health—how we feel both emotionally and physically—hinges on the state of our microbiome."*
>
> —*Dr. David Perlmutter*

**The last decade has been nothing short of a revolution in our** understanding of the role the gut plays in our overall health and wellness. This shake-up in our knowledge about how disease is caused has been spearheaded by an exponential increase in our understanding of the secret world of the microbiome inside each and every one of us.

Our gut's microbiome is like a vast internal galaxy. The bacteria that make up this microbiome outnumber our bodies' cells 10:1 and together contain up to 150 times more genes than our own genome.[1] It is fair to say that our newfound appreciation of the influence these tiny microorganisms have over all aspects of our health truly puts us at the helm of a microbiome revolution.

We are now looking at disease from a new perspective—through the lens of how disturbances in the complex ecosystem of the microbiome trigger or perpetuate all sorts of conditions and diseases, and how rebalancing this system can re-create wellness in your body.

As a medical doctor who specializes in gut health (aka "America's Gut Doctor"), this is my primary focus. I've seen the dramatic impact that an out-of-whack gut can have on your health, mood, and likelihood of developing specific diseases, and how healing the gut can unlock your potential for optimal well-being, happiness, and total body wellness. However, I'm not alone in my enthusiasm. Over the last decade, gut health has gone mainstream as we have learned how the trillions of microbes in our gut impact nearly every disease on the planet. Even the word *microbiome* has risen from obscurity to familiarity for most people.

We're on the cusp of an exciting time in understanding human health. As our mastery of the gut microbiome continues to evolve, it will provide us with an essential piece of the puzzle to solve the obesity epidemic and so many other chronic diseases on the planet. And in this chapter, I'm going to show you how the power of the gut microbiome, when balanced, can be your ally in creating the health and wellness you seek.

For me, this emerging research has been incredibly exciting to watch. (Hey, I'm a science nerd!) After all, understanding how these trillions of microbes that reside in the gut influence human health and illness has been a major interest of mine for over a decade. In this chapter, I wanted to take a deeper dive and share the latest research on how the gut microbiome affects our health, to help you better comprehend why it's so important to pay attention to this hidden world inside each and every one of us.

## UNDERSTANDING THE HUMAN GUT MICROBIOME

At this point, you might be asking, "*Why* are these little critters so vitally important?" After all, some experts call the microbiome our "second genome" and even consider it an accessory endocrine gland, helping to regulate our hormones. Let's dive in and look at what makes the microbiome such a big deal.

Among its many roles, the gut microbiome creates important compounds that impact numerous other systems within the body, from your brain (including learning and memory) to your metabolism. As we saw in the last chapter, research shows that your gut microbes can impact everything from weight gain to acne to neurological health. Animal studies show that once populations of certain bacterial species within an animal's gut have been balanced, those animals even respond better to psychological stress.[2]

The sheer number of these microbes is staggering. As mentioned above, the human body is host to trillions of them, including 500 to 1,000 (estimates vary) different species of bacteria, a few dozen types of yeasts and fungi, an unknown number of viruses, and even parasites and worms. The majority of these microbes reside in the large intestine. However, as you may recall from chapter 1, there are many microbiomes both inside and on the surface of the human body, each of which contains their own unique set of microbes, including on the skin, and in the sinuses, nose, mouth, lungs, and vaginal canal. Collectively, the bacteria, fungi, viruses, parasites, and protozoa *inside the gut* make up the *gut ecosystem*, which we call the **gut microbiome**. Think of it like a rainforest ecosystem, with predators and prey, or as an *internal garden*. Just like a garden, it needs weeding, seeding, and fertilizing to thrive and support our wellness.

Over millennia, as humans have evolved to adapt to our ever-changing environments, these gut "bugs" have evolved along with us. Researchers have found that, among other roles, our "friendly" gut microbes, also called **symbionts,** produce vital nutrients like vitamins K and $B_{12}$, keep up with and adapt to our dietary fiber and sugar consumption, support digestion, play a key role in detoxification, help protect against other gut pathogens, and regulate our immune system by maintaining a healthy gut lining and promoting T regulatory cells (a type of white blood cell that helps keep the immune response from running rampant).[3]

Not all of the gut's microorganisms carry equal weight. Many don't seem to impact health at all. But that doesn't mean they're doing nothing. They may be contributing through an observed effect called **cross-feeding**, where the metabolic byproducts of one type of gut bacteria help support the growth of other beneficial gut bacteria.

A normal gut also harbors unfriendly flora. In fact, 10 to 15 percent of your gut flora would be considered unfavorable microorganisms. Hey, every ecosystem is going to have its mix of villains and helpers! Some of these pathogens, when not held in check by "good" microbes, trigger inflammation (including inflammatory conditions like colitis) and exacerbate many diseases.[4] But that doesn't mean our goal should be to get rid of them entirely. They likely serve yet-to-be-understood roles in improving microbial diversity in the gut, which is the key to wellness.

Sometimes, a bad bug gets into the gut and causes an acute infection characterized by diarrhea, nausea, vomiting, and/or abdominal pain. However, not all gut-related health problems are due to gut infections as we normally think of them, like food poisoning. Many issues arising from the gut are caused by shifts in the delicate balance within the gut ecosystem that happen slowly over time.

### Why Microbiome Diversity Is Important

Okay, pause! Let me briefly explain the importance of gut microbiome diversity, by which I mean the presence of a wide range of species of microorganisms in the gut. **Greater diversity means less inflammation in the gut, as well as the entire body.** The reason has to do with the balance between good and bad bugs. The "good" bacteria produce favorable metabolic byproducts that reduce gut and body-wide inflammation. When diversity is lost, whether due to antibiotics or other factors I will discuss later, the balance shifts. Fewer good bacteria leads to greater inflammation, which is the common root cause for every chronic, degenerative disease.

In summary: **GUT MICROBIAL DIVERSITY = OPTIMAL HEALTH**.

## THE IMPORTANCE OF MICROBIAL BALANCE

The microbiome is a very complex symbiotic system that we are still learning about. What we do know is that balance—in scientific terms, *homeostasis*—is key. In a healthy gut microbiome, the gut bacteria maintain a state of harmony, or *symbiosis*. When the gut microbiome, our gut, and our body are in balance, we can achieve optimal health.

While a healthy gut maintains this balance of good and bad microflora, when that balance is disrupted, it opens the door for unfriendly microbes to step in and take over.

Unfortunately, our good gut bugs are under attack by many aspects of modern life, such as prescription drug use (including antibiotics), environmental toxins and pesticides, GMOs (due to the overuse of glyphosate; I explore this in chapter 5), sleep deprivation, chronic stress, and the use of antibacterial products. Going back to my previous analogy, imagine the delicate biosphere of a rainforest getting taken over by predators—or even worse, deforestation (the equivalent of excess antibiotic use; more on this in chapter 4), which drastically disturbs the ecosystem. When good gut bugs are lost, it opens the terrain for bad bugs to take over.

But nothing creates quite the whammy against gut health as a poor diet. Our ever-adapting gut microbiome has been dramatically altered by the sugary, heavily processed foods that appeared in our food supply in the last fifty or so years. When you eat these foods, it's as if you're choosing to populate your gut with rebels that disrupt the natural state of order within the gut. And by doing so, you're sabotaging your ability to feel great—and lose weight. The Standard American Diet (SAD), which is full of sugar, processed foods, and food additives, actually promotes the growth of harmful bacteria and yeast. In turn, these gut bugs scramble your insulin signaling (more on this to come), leading to weight gain and increased belly fat. Even worse, the SAD is no longer just an American thing—our diet has been exported worldwide, with fast-food chains invading every corner of the globe.

I'll talk about the relationship between dysbiosis of the gut microbiome and your health below. But first, let's look more closely at the diet that best supports gut microbiome diversity.

## THE BEST DIET FOR MICROBIAL DIVERSITY

In the last decade alone, we've learned so much about the gut, the microbiome, the body, and how to eat in ways that support their health. That said, the world of gut health science is fast-paced and constantly changing, with new things uncovered every year. Inevitably, some of those findings contradict what we've previously thought to be true, and so we update our beliefs and recommendations to align with the latest research.

I've seen this happen many times throughout my years of practicing medicine. In fact, as I first sat down to write this book, I read a new piece of evidence—a clinical study done by researchers at the Stanford University School of Medicine—that revealed something surprising about the best diet for gut health.[5] You can imagine my excitement; I couldn't wait to share this with you!

For years, we thought that eating a high-fiber diet was the best way to increase microbial diversity in the gut. But the Stanford study found that while a high-fiber diet did help by improving the way the immune system functions in the long term, *the most dramatic improvements in microbial diversity and inflammatory markers were achieved through a diet high in fermented foods* (at least in the short term).[‡] We're talking sauerkraut, kimchi, pickles, fermented cottage cheese, yogurt, kefir—the works.

Previously, we thought that while fermented foods were a great complement to a gut-friendly diet, a high-fiber diet was the most important way to create diversity in the gut microbiome (the Holy Grail of gut health!). This Stanford study, though, suggests that it's the reverse. It's fermented foods that should be the foundation of a gut-friendly diet (with some caveats I'll discuss in chapter 7), and a high-fiber diet may not be the cure-all for gut health we once thought.

## Fermented foods should be the foundation of a gut-friendly diet.

The picture is more complex than that, and we'll get into more details about how to eat for your gut in the coming chapters. And gut health science is fast-paced and constantly changing (which is why you'll find the most up-to-date information by visiting my blog at **HappyGutLife.com/blog**). But the important message here

---

‡ Note: This was a small, randomized prospective, short (ten-week) dietary intervention study, including only eighteen participants in each diet group, which were mainly composed of white women. It would be great to repeat this study with a larger and more diverse study population, to confirm the effects and see if they can be extrapolated to both men and women, as well as to different ethnicities.

is that a hybrid diet incorporating both fiber-rich and fermented foods is probably the best gut-healthy diet. We'll talk about how to personalize this advice in Part II.

The good news is that with the right foods, you can dramatically improve your gut flora for better gut and immune health, weight management, respiratory health, and much more . . . starting with your very next meal. Your gut flora shifts with dietary changes within just *forty-eight hours*. New research is even showing us *which* foods provide those benefits. One study, for instance, found that eating 43 grams of walnuts daily (about 1.5 ounces or twenty-one walnut halves) for eight weeks significantly enhanced inflammation-busting bacteria within the gut microbiome.[6] I don't know about you, but I certainly want more of those inflammation-busting bacteria hanging around in my gut!

But achieving and maintaining wellness is not just about finding and bingeing on the next superfood. It relies on the sum total of a kaleidoscopic array of foods you consume each week. Making sure that what you choose to put at the end of your fork includes the right combination of key nutrients significantly impacts the health-promoting effects of your gut microbiome.

Unfortunately, when the Standard American Diet, excess alcohol, too much coffee, and lots of sugar prevail in the diet, that's a setup for gut microbiome imbalances that lead to leaky gut and all the diseases associated with it.

Gut health science is fast-paced and constantly changing! You'll find the most up-to-date information by visiting my blog at **HappyGutLife.com/blog**.

## GUT MICROBIOME IMBALANCES, LEAKY GUT, & DISEASE

Our understanding of the gut microbiome is still in its infancy,[7] but here's what we know for sure: Imbalances in the gut flora influence gut permeability (or "leakiness") and create chaos not only in the gut, but in the rest of the body as well, contributing to or exacerbating many health problems that plague modern-day society. Over the past few years, studies have shown how gut dysbiosis plays a role in obesity, diabetes, cancer, and many other diseases. In the coming years, I believe emerging studies will continue to elucidate how gut health impacts these and other diseases.

Before we look at this fascinating research, I want to emphasize that many of these conditions are *multifactorial* problems. In other words, they are the result of the sum total of many triggers—lack of sleep, chronic stress, side effects from prescription drugs (especially antibiotics), and poor nutrition (particularly a diet devoid of enough fiber and fermented foods) among them—that can either lead to dysbiosis or affect these diseases directly. As I'll explain, however, we cannot underestimate the impact your gut health has on these conditions, or on your overall state of well-being. Gut microbiome imbalances, including their effect on gut permeability that inevitably leads to leaky gut and inflammation, are a surprising driving factor in a number of health issues—including obesity, insulin resistance and diabetes, metabolic syndrome, and risk for heart disease and stroke.

Emerging research suggests that the hidden world of your microbiota actually is the master puppeteer when it comes to maintaining a healthy weight. And just like in puppetry, we may be fooled into thinking the puppet (our body) is moving itself, when it's actually the puppeteer (our microbiome) that is pulling the strings. The gut microbiome responds to diet, antibiotics, and other external stimuli quickly, with precision, and in ways that impact and can even control a variety of metabolic conditions.[8]

Let's look at several of these related conditions in detail.

## The Gut Microbiome & Obesity

The latest research is refuting the decades-held belief that weight loss and weight maintenance are controlled by the simple difference between calories in and calories out. Body composition is more nuanced than that, and the gut microbiome plays a significant role. A number of studies have associated obesity with altered gut microbiota; for example, researchers find that in both humans and rodents, lean and overweight subjects differ in the composition of their intestinal flora.[9]

Obesity and its characteristic alterations in the composition and function of the human gut microbiome seem to feed off each other (pardon the pun) in a vicious cycle: The release of inflammatory molecules associated with obesity perpetuates bad gut flora, which in turn provoke more inflammation that can stall your weight loss efforts.[10]

But this is not the only way gut imbalances can impact your weight. Cross-sectional studies show that gut microbes can influence your body's ability to extract and store calories.[11] And this, in turn, plays a significant role in determining your body composition and weight. As with other conditions I'll discuss, the wrong type of microbial "map" (that is, microbial composition) or *lack of diversity* can set the stage for obesity and hold your weight hostage in a never-ending weight loss plateau. What this means is that investing in *your gut health is the answer to resistant weight loss and maintaining a healthy weight.*

## Making Thin Mice Fat, Then Thin Again

Recent mind-blowing research studies have looked at how altering gut flora can impact weight. In one such study, scientists took the gut microbes from four sets of identical human twins in which one twin was slim and the other obese and transferred them into two groups of mice that had been raised in a germ-free environment (so their bodies *and guts* would be free of any bacteria).[12]

The researchers found that the mice given microbes from an obese twin quickly gained weight, whereas the mice populated with microbes from a lean twin stayed thin. To factor out any differences in eating patterns as the reason for the weight gain, both sets of mice were given the same diet. It was the clearest evidence to date that gut bacteria can cause obesity.

The researchers then looked at whether obesity could be reversed simply by increasing the diversity of gut microbial populations. The thin mice were placed in the same cage with the obese mice, and as a result of their commingling, the more-diverse microbiota from the lean mice transferred to and took over the gut of their obese cage mates, who had started with a less-diverse population. (This is the equivalent of a **fecal transplant** in humans—the process of transferring fecal bacteria from a healthy individual into a sick individual, via an enema or capsules.) As hoped, this one-way transfer resulted in an improved metabolism and a reversal of obesity in the obese mice . . . as long as all the mice were fed a low-fat diet.

When, in a follow-up experiment, the formerly obese mice were fed a diet high in saturated fats, they gained weight again and their gut flora reverted to a less diverse makeup. The study also showed that, once obese, the mice lost the ability to lose weight and correct metabolic abnormalities when fed a high-fat diet—even when cohabiting with thin mice. In other words, the gut of the obese mice was colonized with the healthier gut flora of the thin mice, resulting in weight loss and metabolic improvements, *only* when they were fed a diet low in saturated fat and high in fruits and vegetables. As these experiments show, you have to feed your microbiome the right diet to maintain that diversity and promote weight loss.[13] You can't stay thin while having your cake and eating it, too!

One meta-analysis looked at the structural and functional changes of the gut microbiota in rodents that were fed a high-fat diet until they became obese. Researchers found that the high-fat diet induced changes in their gut microbial composition that were associated with obesity. This altered gut microbiome triggered and promoted *insulin resistance* (explained below) and systemic inflammation, the root causes for weight gain in the majority of people.[14]

Animal-model obesity studies, like human ones, keep pointing back to the same idea: that **the inciting factor in weight gain is the gut microbiome**.

If the underlying problem in obesity is the gut microbiome, why don't we just use fecal transplants to make obese people thin again? Unfortunately, human studies have struggled to identify the exact microbial "map" that translates into obesity. But some potential causes have surfaced.

Mouse experiments have looked at the ratio of two important groups of bacteria that seem to play a strong role in metabolism: *Firmicutes* and *Bacteroidetes*. Some scientists have suggested that a high ratio of *Firmicutes* to *Bacteroidetes* correlates with a greater propensity toward obesity and could be used as a biomarker for it; however, using this ratio as a hallmark for obesity has yielded contradictory results.[15] We're not quite there yet. The ability to manipulate gut flora to affect weight in humans is not as straightforward as it may seem, based on the mouse experiments described above. Thus far, attempts to pinpoint which bacterial species are responsible for a normal body mass have been inconclusive.

The truth is that the gut microbiome is a very complex, symbiotic system that is influenced by lifestyle and dietary factors, as well as yet-to-be-discovered bacterial species that affect microbial diversity and composition in ways that we are still elucidating. And as the percentage of processed foods in our diets has increased over the last century and the use of antibiotics has skyrocketed, the microbial populations in the human gut have become less and less diverse. We are literally causing an epidemic of gut and gut-related illnesses through our lifestyle choices. What we *do* know is that the right, personalized diet (like the one outlined in the GutSMART Protocol) can optimize and diversify our gut microflora, improving overall health and leading to sometimes rapid and sustained weight loss, even for people who have been stuck on a weight loss plateau for years.

## The Gut Microbiome, Insulin Resistance & Diabetes

**Insulin** is the body's critical blood sugar–regulating hormone. **Insulin resistance** occurs when your body requires more insulin to maintain a steady level of sugar circulating in your bloodstream because your cells "resist" this hormone's signal. It's as if the cells in your body become deaf to insulin's signal, so your pancreas needs to turn up the volume (that is, secrete more insulin) for your cells to "hear" it. This overproduction of insulin leads to unwanted fat accumulation around the middle, weight gain, obesity, and eventually, over the course of many years, type 2 diabetes.

Insulin resistance is especially dangerous because it ramps up the persistent low-grade inflammation caused by chronic activation of the immune system.[16] And as we've discussed, chronic inflammation is the key driver behind pretty much every known disease.

Why am I talking about insulin resistance in a chapter about the gut microbiome? It's because the microbiome holds the key to how we process sugar.

For years, it was commonly believed that insulin resistance was caused by eating too many simple starches, sugars, and artificial sweeteners. What we didn't realize until recently is the role the gut microbiome plays, by controlling nutrient

## INSULIN RESISTANCE

Gut microbes exert control over insulin sensitivity and resistance. Good gut bacteria increase insulin sensitivity, while bad gut bacteria scramble the insulin signal, leading to insulin resistance at the insulin receptor. As a result, the pancreas secretes too much insulin. It is as if the cells become deaf to the insulin signal, so your body needs to turn up the volume for your cells to "hear" it.

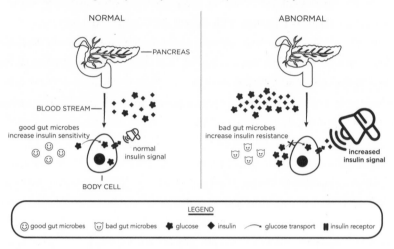

availability and in regulating our blood sugar and sensitivity to the insulin signal. Research shows that gut microbiota play a major role in several factors that may lead to insulin resistance: the extraction of energy from the foods we eat, the maintenance of proper gut barrier function, and the control of body inflammation, all of which influence the development of both obesity and diabetes.[17] When your microbiome becomes dysbiotic and your gut leaky, it can scramble the insulin signal, leading to insulin resistance and all the problems it ushers in, including eventually type 2 diabetes.

### How the Microbiome Affects Insulin Sensitivity

A healthy body is maintained through the internal balance between our gut microflora and the metabolic byproducts they secrete, collectively referred to as the **metabolome.** The key metabolites (or **postbiotics**) produced by gut microbiota are **short-chain fatty acids** (SCFAs), one of the most important of which is *butyrate*.

These SCFAs are the primary energy source for colon cells. They also impact insulin signaling, blood sugar regulation, neuroplasticity in the brain, and something called the *inflammatory cascade*, in which an initial immune reaction (to an infection, for example) leads to an outpouring of other inflammatory signals.[18] When the microbes in your gut aren't producing enough SCFAs because of a dysbiosis, your gut lining becomes more permeable, inflammatory signals increase, insulin resistance increases, and even learning, memory, and mental health can be affected. Consuming a diet high in fiber, like the one outlined in the GutSMART Protocol in chapter 7, gives your gut bacteria the nutrients it needs to create more of these beneficial SCFAs.

Worldwide, type 2 diabetes currently affects about 400 million people. By 2035, this number is expected to jump to 600 million. The problem is most doctors don't check for insulin resistance, which can precede diabetes by up to a decade. Once they find diabetes, it's often too late to reverse the process. But years before diabetes sets in, metabolic syndrome plays in the background, often ignored or undiagnosed until it's too late.

## The Gut Microbiome & Metabolic Syndrome

**Metabolic syndrome** is a condition characterized by weight gain, elevated blood sugar levels, elevated triglycerides, low HDL ("good" cholesterol), and increased belly fat that can eventually lead to type 2 diabetes. As with most diseases in Western medicine, this condition is named based on the constellation of findings it is characterized by rather than its root cause. Sometimes this is because we aren't yet sure of the root cause. With metabolic syndrome, we are: *Metabolic syndrome is the result of insulin resistance*, which can be rooted in a dysbiotic gut microbiome and leaky gut.

*Why is metabolic syndrome so important?* Along with obesity and diabetes, it is a *major* driving factor for many other diseases, including nonalcoholic fatty liver disease, cardiovascular disorders (like high blood pressure, heart attacks, and stroke), neurodegenerative diseases, and several types of cancer.[19] Metabolic syndrome is also a major cause of heart attacks and vascular diseases. In fact, it may be *more* dangerous for heart health than diabetes because it can go unnoticed for years, as high insulin levels (due to insulin resistance) wreak havoc on the circulatory system. During those years, blood pressure rises and plaque builds up inside the arterial walls, eventually leading to blockages in the coronary arteries of the heart.

### The Gut Microbiome & Heart Disease

Metabolic syndrome isn't the only way the gut microbiome impacts heart health. It turns out that gut bacteria can also produce a molecule known as **trimethylamine** (**TMA**), which gets absorbed into the bloodstream. When processed by the liver into **TMAO** (**trimethylamine N-oxide**), it doubles the risk of heart attack and stroke—regardless of the presence of other risk factors like smoking, high blood pressure, and metabolic syndrome.

As it turns out, TMA is made when gut bacteria process food nutrients like L-carnitine from red meat and phosphatidylcholine from shellfish. When that TMA passes through the liver and is converted to TMAO, then released into the circulation, it can in turn lead to platelet activation, contribute to plaque formation, and cause tiny blood clots in the heart and brain as a result. *The takeaway?* If you want to reduce your potential for TMAO production and cut your risk for heart disease and stroke, cut back on red meat and shellfish—and eat more veggies, which have been shown to lower TMA production.

## WHO'S REALLY IN CHARGE?

> *"Am I simply a vehicle for numerous bacteria that inhabit my microbiome? Or are they hosting me?"*
>
> —Timothy Morton

Remember that analogy of the puppet and the puppeteer? Who is really pulling the strings here—you or your microbiome? The more we learn, the more we realize the gut microbiome is in charge of maintaining important levels of homeostasis within the body.

Other factors also come into play, of course, but alterations in the gut microbiota (from modern advances like antibiotics and environmental chemicals, poor diet, poor sleep, or mental stress) have become the major driver of insulin resistance, metabolic syndrome, and their related conditions. Most notably, these factors include the reduction of circulating SCFAs like butyrate, which then lowers insulin sensitivity and increases the risk for obesity.[20]

The good news is that insulin resistance, like all the health problems discussed in chapter 2—as detrimental and systemic as they can become—are also potentially reversible by balancing your gut microbiome with the dietary and lifestyle factors I discuss later in this book.

A diverse gut flora is the key to wellness, and what you will learn in the next chapter are the key factors impacting microbial diversity in your gut. So, if you're serious about improving the health of your gut flora, come dive with me into some of the biggest threats to gut health. Let's go!

## Takeaways

There are many important takeaways in this chapter... but if there's only one thing you remember from it, remember this:
**GUT MICROBIOME DIVERSITY = OPTIMAL HEALTH**.

1.  Your gut microbiome is a complex ecosystem.

2.  Poor diet (along with other factors discussed in the next chapter) cause gut microbiome imbalances or *dysbiosis*, leading to leaky gut. This is causing an epidemic of gut and gut-related illnesses worldwide.

3.  When you choose the right combination of key nutrients to put at the end of your fork, you can significantly impact the healthfulness of your gut microbiome.

4.  Eating fermented foods is a key part of the strategy for promoting gut microbial diversity and reducing body-wide inflammation.

5. The gut microbiome plays a much greater role in controlling nutrient availability, regulating our blood sugar, and determining our sensitivity to the insulin signal than we previously appreciated.

6. Gut microbiome imbalances are the driving factor in a number of conditions, including obesity, insulin resistance and diabetes, metabolic syndrome, and heart disease.

7. Your gut health is the answer to resistant weight loss and maintaining a healthy weight.

8. When the microbes in your gut aren't producing enough SCFAs because of a dysbiosis, gut permeability increases, inflammatory signals increase, insulin resistance increases, and even learning, memory, and mental health can be affected.

Chapter 4

# THE BIGGEST THREATS
# TO GUT HEALTH

*"We spent an enormous amount of time . . .
living as hunter-gatherers. . . . We're suddenly
living in this profoundly unnatural way, and
we're still in the process of adapting to it."*

—Spencer Wells

**In February 2020, I had the opportunity to experience what it** might have been like to be alive thousands of years ago. I was one of a select group of twelve people that were invited to go meet and live with the Hadza in East Africa—one of the last groups of hunter-gatherers on the planet—for three days and two nights. No trip has defined my life as a gut health expert and functional medicine practitioner more than this trip to Africa. It was truly a way to go back to *the roots of digestion* and understand our relationship to the world around us before we altered it through technology and modern sanitation practices. I knew this trip would be important in expanding my understanding of human health, but I had no idea how much my time with the Hadza would illuminate for me the biggest threats to gut health.

To give you a little background, the Hadza are a modern hunter-gatherer tribe of about 1,000 members residing in northern Tanzania, known not only for being one of the last remaining groups of hunter-gatherers on Earth but also for being extraordinarily healthy. Prior to the trip, I was aware of a number of studies that had been done on the Hadza people and their gut microbiomes, so I wanted to see for myself the kind of lifestyle they lead. Two years prior, at a microbiome conference, I had been to a lecture by a scientist who had lived with the Hadza. He presented how the Hadza were free of the scourge of modern disease. They had no diabetes, no heart disease, no cancer, no dementia, and no obesity while living a primitive existence. Do they still get respiratory infections, like bronchitis? Absolutely, yes! But, as the tribal chief revealed to me during my own visit, while they have no modern medicines like antibiotics, they use secret herbal remedies handed down to them by their elders. My curiosity was piqued.

During my trip, I went hunting and gathering with them, foraging for root vegetables and even eating them raw, freshly dug out of the earth. We went into the bush, tracked down a beehive hidden inside a tree's bark, and got to sample fresh, raw honey, eating the honeycomb and even the tiny live African bees that got mixed in with the honey. Before you cringe at the thought of eating honeybees, know that they looked more like tiny flies than bees. It's not something I'd ever done before, but I thought, *Hey, when in Tanzania, do as the Hadza do*. So I stretched out my hand and watched the tribe member pour raw, fresh honey, mixed with all those things, into it. I'd never felt more connected with the earth, with where our food comes from, and where we as humans fit into that picture, than on that day.

The Hadza people have a unique and specific diet made up of the seasonal and regional foods they're able to hunt or gather where they live. They primarily eat root vegetables (tubers), berries, wild honey, baobab fruit, and small- to medium-size game animals. Much to my dismay, though they eat a diet rich in fiber, they don't "eat the rainbow"—a concept we teach and preach in functional medicine as a necessity for health and wellness—and in spite of that, they have a more diverse gut microbiome than people in the West (aka you and me), based on an age-matched Italian control group.[1] Even more surprising, the Italian study showed that the Hadza's gut microbiomes are even more diverse than those of people following a Mediterranean diet—one of the healthiest diets on the planet.[2]

This made me rethink my view of gut health and microbiome diversity, and allowed me to open my mind to a greater understanding of what *really* creates optimal gut health. The whole experience underscored how profoundly our connection to the earth and exposure to soil can improve our gut health. Unlike Western societies, there's a lack of basic hygiene among the Hadza people. You won't see them washing their hands or using antibacterial soaps or hand sanitizers. And yet, despite this, they are among the healthiest people on the planet.

So why *do* the Hadza have more diverse gut microbiomes and less disease than the Western, "civilized" world? I think there are several reasons:

- Lack of exposure to antibiotics
- Consumption of large amounts of gut microbiome–supportive fiber
- Greater exposure to positive stressors like the elements (which do not kill you but make you stronger; more on this in the next chapter) and less exposure to negative stressors like chronic mental stress (more on this in chapter 10)
- Lack of excessive cleanliness and exposure to the microbiome of the soil, which enhances gut microbiome diversity

In the previous chapters, we discussed the gut, the microbiome, and all of the symptoms, diseases, and conditions that can stem from damage to them. We've also discussed the connection between dysbiosis and leaky gut—the root cause of the majority of chronic health conditions—and how everything in the body is connected to the gut in some way, shape, or form. But my experience with the Hadza poignantly highlighted some of the biggest factors threatening our gut microbial biodiversity. In the rest of this chapter and the next, I want to look at these one at a time, beginning with the *Western healthcare system*, and specifically antibiotics.

## THE GUT-HARMING EFFECTS OF ANTIBIOTICS

As an MD who has worked in the medical field for over two decades, I have seen firsthand how rampant the overprescribing of medications is—and in particular, how overprescribed antibiotics are. The Centers for Disease Control (CDC) has found that at least 30 percent of antibiotics prescribed in the United States are unnecessary.[3] When you run the numbers, that comes out to 47 million excess antibiotic prescriptions per year!

Even more concerning is the fact that in a large number of countries, antibiotics can be purchased from a pharmacy without a prescription from a doctor. In Europe alone, twenty-eight countries allow the sale of antibiotics without a prescription,[4] and not surprisingly, the sales and usage of antibiotics continue to multiply. This overuse of antibiotics has led to the development of *superbugs*, with antibiotic resistance rising worldwide.[5] (I'll discuss this further in a few pages.)

Antibiotics, as you may already know, are used to treat infections in the body caused by bacteria. They are quite effective at doing this. In fact, when used appropriately, antibiotics save lives. I saw this as a doctor-in-training at the hospital and have repeatedly helped keep patients out of the hospital *by prescribing the right antibiotic at the right time*. The problem is that antibiotics don't just kill off harmful, infection-causing bacteria. They also kill off good bacteria—specifically good bacteria in your gut. When your gut is wiped of its resident good bacteria, the microbiome becomes imbalanced. This dysbiosis, as discussed in chapter 1, contributes to a whole host of gut-related issues, like constipation, diarrhea, leaky gut, gas, bloating, nausea, and yeast overgrowth or infection, to name a few.[6]

Your gut doesn't just bounce back right after taking a course of antibiotics. For example, a five-day course of ciprofloxacin (sold under the brand name Cipro)—an antibiotic of the fluoroquinolone class commonly given to women to treat urinary tract infections—causes a dysbiosis that can take up to twelve months to resolve.[7] Another commonly prescribed antibiotic, azithromycin (best known as Zithromax or the five-day "Z-Pak")—used to treat a variety of upper respiratory infections, including COVID-19—can lead to a six-month-long dysbiosis.[8]

I was shocked to find out how long dysbiosis can last after taking antibiotics—despite having had it happen to me. As you might remember from my gut-healing journey, when I was ten years old, I started getting sick frequently. I had lots of infections: throat infections, sinus infections, respiratory infections—you name it, I had it. During the seven years that followed, I spent hours and hours in doctors' offices, and was put on antibiotic after antibiotic, but these medicines just seemed to make my health even worse. At the time, I thought I was born with a weak immune system and that I was more susceptible than others to getting sick—I had become a teenage hypochondriac, constantly worried I would get ill from being exposed to a sick person or harmful bacteria, struggling to stay healthy. I kept asking myself over and over: *Why am I constantly getting sick?* What neither I nor my parents or pediatricians knew then was that the constant antibiotics were a fundamental part of the problem. And I want to share with you what I know now in the hope that I can keep you from falling prey to the same vicious cycle that left me fighting to feel well for the next two decades of my life.

## How Antibiotics Destroyed My Gut

From the age of ten through the end of my teenage years, I was on antibiotics *two or three times a year*, which is a lot by any doctor's standards. Sometimes I was even given gamma globulin shots (shots that temporarily boost your immunity by giving you pooled antibodies from people who have donated blood) because the doctor said my immune system was so weak I wasn't responding to the antibiotics I was prescribed. I was also prescribed multivitamins and told first to lose weight (when I was a chubby ten-year-old), then to gain weight (when I stretched out after my teenage growth spurt between ages twelve and thirteen and became super thin), but as it turns out, neither vitamins nor my weight had anything to do with the problem.

The real issue was that my gut microbiome was repeatedly being decimated by antibiotics, which consequently weakened my immune system. This resulted in a whole host of health problems, including irritable bowel syndrome, leaky gut, migraines, mental fog, and skin rashes.

Thankfully, as I got older, I stopped getting sick as often—sometimes through accidental changes in my diet, like cutting out most of the dairy and incorporating more healthy fats when I went to medical school at the age of twenty-one. That meant I wasn't taking as many antibiotics, which gave my gut a chance to start healing. It took a lot of time and effort to fully heal, though, because medical school didn't offer a clear perspective on how nutrition affects our bodies. In fact, diet and nutrition maybe got an honorable mention during one of my med school courses (when they should have—at a minimum—gotten their own year-long course). Since then, I have dedicated my life and my professional work to learning about and understanding gut health and nutrition, and about how eating well can rebalance the gut microbiome and reverse leaky gut. And you better believe I'm not rampantly prescribing pointless antibiotics to my patients!

## The Dangers of Excessive Antibiotics

I'm certainly not completely anti-antibiotics. There are instances where antibiotics are necessary, and it's a medical miracle that we can clear up infections that centuries ago would have killed us en masse. When I caution against antibiotics, my point is that **not every single infection requires antibiotics**. In fact, there are thousands (and probably millions) of cases where antibiotics are prescribed for infections they're incapable of curing!

The CDC found that most unnecessary antibiotics are prescribed to treat respiratory infections caused by viruses like the common cold, viral sore throats, bronchitis, and sinus and ear infections.[9] For the most common childhood infection, acute otitis media of the ear, a pediatrician prescribing antibiotics has traditionally been as predictable as suggesting you need to drink water when you sweat. But according to the American Academy of Family Physicians, antibiotics are often overused in children for these ear infections, and it's possible for children to recover just fine without them.[10] These ailments by and large don't require antibiotics because antibiotics are meant to treat bacterial infections, not viral ones, and most of these infections are actually caused by viruses. When you use antibiotics to try to treat a viral infection, you're essentially devastating the population of healthy bacteria in your gut for no reason and potentially triggering unpleasant symptoms in other parts of your body as a result. And it's important to remember that what is done to you in childhood can play a very significant role in your health as an adult.

Studies have shown the long-term impact that childhood antibiotics have on the gut, and they underscore how imbalances in the gut can cause issues in the rest of the body. For example, one study found that disruptions in the gut caused by antibiotics early in life can affect metabolism and increase a person's risk of impaired growth, weight gain, and obesity.[11] Subsequent studies have affirmed this, finding that the use of antibiotics early in life is associated with an increased risk of metabolic and immune diseases.[12]

Furthermore, antibiotics not only decimate the gut flora, they also affect the health of the lining of the small intestine, leading to increased intestinal permeability and the reduced production of digestive enzymes. This can cause serious issues because, as you may recall, a leaky gut, combined with food that is not well broken down due to a lack of digestive enzymes, can lead to food reactions and sensitivities. And once this cascade of events happens, weight gain, headaches or

## ANTIBIOTIC RESISTANCE

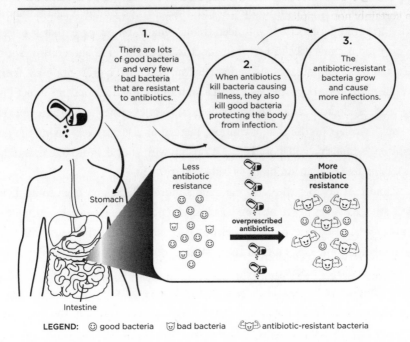

**1.**
There are lots of good bacteria and very few bad bacteria that are resistant to antibiotics.

**2.**
When antibiotics kill bacteria causing illness, they also kill good bacteria protecting the body from infection.

**3.**
The antibiotic-resistant bacteria grow and cause more infections.

Stomach

Less antibiotic resistance

overprescribed antibiotics

More antibiotic resistance

Intestine

**LEGEND:** ☺ good bacteria ☺ bad bacteria ☺ antibiotic-resistant bacteria

migraines, skin rashes, mental fog, fatigue, and irritable bowel syndrome tend to follow, until eventually, you may even develop an autoimmune disease.

Perhaps worst of all, the overprescribing of antibiotics can cause the bacteria in our bodies to become antibiotic resistant, meaning any bacteria antibiotics don't manage to wipe out can adapt and develop defense mechanisms against future antibiotics.[13] In other words, the infection-causing bacteria become harder to kill, so doctors have to prescribe stronger or higher doses of antibiotics to fight infections. Then the cycle repeats.[14] Eventually, antibiotics become useless, and infections either get to a point where they have progressed beyond treatment, or you are forced to resort to less reliable and effective treatment methods.

To sum it up, the overuse of antibiotics puts you, me, and everyone else who is needlessly prescribed them (or buys them over the counter, like in countries that allow the purchase of antibiotics without a doctor's prescription) at risk for allergic reactions, deadly diarrhea, and a host of chronic gut-related health problems.

## What You Can Do

*Don't take unnecessary antibiotics.* I said it before, and I'll say it again: I am *not* saying to avoid antibiotics if you need them. What I *am* saying is that it pays to have a candid conversation with your doctor about the pros and cons of antibiotics and research potential side effects before accepting a prescription. Ask this one question: "Do you *really* feel I need an antibiotic to knock out this infection?" The truth is, doctors are often prescribing antibiotics either to appease you (the patient) or to err on the side of caution. Instead of just passively taking the prescription, establish a collaborative relationship with your doctor so that together you can figure out if an antibiotic is truly right for you.

I find that doctors who, like me, take a more holistic approach to medicine that's still grounded in science are less likely to prescribe *unnecessary* antibiotics. So my biggest piece of advice is to seek out a doctor who has experience with functional medicine and make it clear to them that you want to take antibiotics only if they are *absolutely necessary.*

It's important to take back your power as a patient and co-creator of your own health. And one of the most powerful ways you can do that, the one that is the focus of this book, is something you do every single day, when you pick up a fork or spoon. *You are making a conscious choice about what you put in your mouth to nourish your body.*

# GUT HEALTH & YOUR FOOD CHOICES

In the last chapter, we touched on the best dietary choices for gut and overall health. But beyond avoiding excess red meat and shellfish and eating more fiber-rich veggies and fermented foods, does the type of food you eat matter? Should you care if your food is organic or not? Does it matter where the meats you eat came from, and what those animals ate? How about the conditions under which they were raised? If there were hormones or antibiotics in the feed? What about the conditions under which the fruits and vegetables you eat were grown, and whether they were sprayed with pesticides? How about the additives and preservatives in the processed food you eat?

The simple answer to these questions is an emphatic *yes*! When you focus on eating foods that are organic, pesticide-free, and non-GMO—with bonus points for foods that are locally grown and sustainably farmed—you not only make a difference in the environment and support your local growers (more on this in the next chapter), but, most importantly for our purposes, also promote your overall health by supporting your gut microbiome.

While these foods might cost a little more or occasionally be more challenging to find, I absolutely believe that choosing the highest-quality foods—if and when you can—has a dramatic impact on your gut.

## The most important factor in gut health that you have personal control over is your diet.

You may be wondering, *Does the cost justify eating organic? Is it really healthier?* The research says *yes*! Multiple studies have shown that organic foods contain significantly higher amounts of vitamins and nutrients, including vitamin C, folate, iron, magnesium, and phosphorus, than nonorganic varieties of the same foods. Organic foods are also significantly lower in nitrates (a harmful ingredient found in synthetic fertilizers and often used as a chemical preservative in cured meats) and pesticide residues and contain higher amounts of antioxidants compared to nonorganic versions.[15] I see this in the produce I buy from my local organic farmer—without a doubt, it stays fresher for longer in my refrigerator. That's the power of a higher antioxidant load and freshly picked produce!

Buying quality animal foods also supports gut health. Several studies suggest grass-fed animal meat contains higher amounts of nutrients and antioxidants and has an overall superior (more heart-healthy and anti-inflammatory) fat profile when compared to grain-fed animals.[16]

This may seem like a lot to take into account because we're not as close to where our food comes from as the Hadza are, but it's really about returning to eating more naturally from the Earth. When we feel more connected with the source of our food, we tend to eat healthier, less processed foods. Children who are taught to grow vegetables in a garden tend to eat more veggies.

Making the right choices for your gut in our modern world takes a bit more knowledge and discernment than just eating what the Earth has to offer, however, which is why, in Part II, we'll look in detail at the foods to eat to help you heal your gut, restore balance to your gut microbiome, and reverse or prevent leaky gut. Gut health also isn't one-size-fits-all—that's why my 14-day GutSMART Protocol, based on your GutSMART Quiz score, is designed to help you personalize the right eating plan for you. With your GutSMART Score in hand, you'll know what food list(s) to follow and which meal plan is best suited for your gut's needs. For now, the key thing to know is that your diet is the means by which to achieve a healthy and diversified gut ecosystem, and therefore your overall best health.

## STRESS & YOUR GUT

As important as what you eat is—and it's very important; that's why it's the center-piece of this book!—diet alone will only get you so far if you live a stressed-out life.

When I sat down with the Hadza tribe chief, one thing that struck me was his cheerful nature and temperament; he didn't seem to take anything too seriously. Even with a language barrier (neither of us understood each other), we managed to communicate through intonation, hand motions, and acting things out with laughter and smiles. It was like a game of charades. But through our translator, I learned the Hadza *do not have a word for depression*. They live with the elements and don't think of adversity as a source of stress; instead, it is the fuel for build-ing their resilience. No wonder they've managed to keep their tribal traditions for thousands of years!

As we'll get into in Part IV, the psychological stress most Western people live under has a dramatic and measurable negative impact on the gut. In fact, I like to say that **stress is like an attack on your gut**. Studies show the hormone surge triggered by the "fight or flight" stress response can alter the natural balance of healthy bac-teria in your gut, inducing a shift in the gut ecology in favor of more hostile groups of bacteria. That's why, as we'll discuss in more detail in chapter 10, managing stress is a crucial component of the GutSMART Protocol. Exercise, optimal sleep, medita-tion, breathing, gratitude, and a positive mental outlook are just as important as any dietary and supplement advice when it comes to creating a healthy, happy gut in a happy body and mind. As much as we can't bypass the right nutrition when healing the gut, we also can't overlook working on our mental and spiritual well-being. But by eating the right foods for your gut type and reducing your stress response, you'll set yourself up for the greatest healing in the shortest amount of time.

## The Hadzas & Resilient Wellness

Regardless of how distant we may feel from the modern-day Hadzas, hunting and gathering in the African bush, we can learn a bunch by peeking into this human time capsule. As much as technology and the world around us have evolved, there's a lot that has stayed constant about what we, and our gut microbiome, need to build resilient wellness. Whereas modern remedies like antibiotics have helped lengthen our lifespan, they have come with a price, because they affect us all the way down to the microscopic level of our microbiome. The smallest things—from the medications we take to what we eat for breakfast to whether we make time for meditation—can have the biggest impact on our health.

But there's another lesson we can take from the Hadza: We are as much a product of the environment in which we live as they are. And that's what we'll turn to in the next chapter.

## Takeaways

Reducing your exposure to antibiotics, eating the right foods personalized for your gut type, and minimizing your stress translate into a richer, more diverse gut microbiome that creates a more robust, resilient immune system, body, and mind.

1.  Antibiotics are gut-disrupting, leading to a loss in gut microbial diversity.

2.  Avoid taking antibiotics unless they are absolutely necessary. Especially avoid taking them to "knock out a cold" or upper respiratory infection, since those illnesses are most often caused by viruses that mostly don't respond to antibiotics anyway.

3.  If you are prescribed an antibiotic, have a real conversation with your doctor and be aware of potential side effects before taking it.

4.  If you have been exposed to multiple rounds of antibiotics throughout your lifetime, you'll need a whole lot of gut-healing.

5.   The most important factor in gut health that you have personal control over is your diet.

6.   What you put at the end of your fork significantly impacts the health effects your gut microbiome has on the rest of your body.

7.   Eat organic produce whenever possible. It's higher in antioxidants and nutrients than nonorganic produce.

8.   Stress is like an attack on your gut. Don't write it off as unimportant—or something you can't do anything about. (See Part IV for more on stress and the best ways to manage it.)

# Chapter 5

# ENVIRONMENTAL THREATS TO GUT HEALTH

> *"Our gut microbiome is a direct extension of the nature that we touch."*
>
> —Dr. Zach Bush

**When we talk about our health, we usually talk about it in terms** that are relative to the body. We talk about the organs and the biological systems and processes that happen inside us, both voluntary and involuntary. But the factors that affect our health aren't confined to what happens inside our bodies; we do not exist in a vacuum. The environment we live in and the soil our food is grown in play a major role in our health, and in particular, the health of our gut microbiome. Now, it's time to zoom out and look at how our gut health is connected to the outside world—specifically, how the soil, biodiversity, and the soil microbiome shape, affect, and can even save your health.

# IT'S NOT JUST ABOUT YOU (EVERYTHING IS INTERCONNECTED)

In the same way that your gut microbiome is connected to every part of your body, there's also a strong connection between your gut and the world around you. In chapter 1, I used the metaphor of a tree to show how the gut is like the root system of the body—how everything that happens in our body starts in the gut. I talked about how if the leaves of a tree look diseased or discolored, you wouldn't try to fix them by painting them green—the equivalent of masking symptoms by taking a drug for them rather than finding and correcting the underlying cause. Instead, you'd look at the tree's root system and the soil it's planted in to figure out what's *really* going on. In the human body, our "root system" is the gut. And in the outside world, as Maria Rodale, granddaughter of J. I. Rodale (who is credited with founding the organic movement), once told me when I had the opportunity to meet with her:

"The soil is like the guts of the earth." —Maria Rodale

That poignant phrase stuck with me after that short meeting years ago. I kept going back to what she said, thinking it was such a beautiful parallel for the connection between the soil and *our* guts. It also serves to remind us of how gut health extends far beyond what is physically happening to the gut inside our bodies at any singular moment—it's so much bigger than that, as I described through my experience with the Hadza. And this is why I feel so passionate about the content I'm going to share with you in this chapter.

## THE IMPORTANCE OF DIVERSITY

A central principle I have repeatedly spoken about since the publishing of my first book, *Happy Gut*, is this simple phrase: **Diversity is the key to sustained wellness.** And by diversity, I mean diversity in so many elements of our lives—diversity in our diet, in our activities, in our positive daily habits. But for the sake of this chapter, what I'm specifically talking about here is diversity as it pertains to the gut microbiome.

*Microbial diversity* is one of the most important concepts that has come out of the gut health movement. As we discussed in chapter 3, the more diverse your gut microbiome is, the healthier you are. In other words, the diversity of your gut microbiome is the yardstick with which to measure your susceptibility to and likelihood of developing disease.

Microbial diversity in the gut helps the body in countless ways: It helps us build immunity, keeps our blood sugar balanced, and allows us to think more clearly.

This is why, when working on healing the gut, one of our main focuses is increasing microbial diversity. But where does this diversity come from? When we are but fetuses in the womb, our guts are primarily sterile environments. It's during the birthing process that we are first "inoculated" with microbes, as we come into contact with the microbiome in our mother's vaginal canal. (This natural process is an important benefit of giving birth vaginally—if possible—rather than by C-section, and why some ob-gyns are starting to "vaginally seed" C-section babies by wiping their face, mouth, and bodies with their mother's vaginal fluids. This process transfers vaginal microbes to the baby, helping to begin the process of establishing a healthy microbiome that is otherwise missed in birth by C-section.) Thereafter, the growth of the first main health-enhancing gut bacteria—*Bifidobacterium infantis*—is supported by the *human milk oligosaccharides* or sugars in breast milk. Holding babies skin-to-skin also reinforces the colonization of the body with the unique microbiome of the skin. And ongoing contact with the outside world continues a baby's microbial "education" until, between the ages of three and five, their microbiome starts looking more like the adult gut microbiome.

While it seems that our gut microbiota are most influenced by environmental factors in the first decade of our lives,[1] we know that our environment shapes our gut microbiome and consequently influences our health in many ways no matter how old we are. What we are coming to realize is that our gut microbiome is more connected to the biodiversity of our planet than previously appreciated.

Gut health is not just about you, the individual. It's about what's happening outside of you, as well.

## BIODIVERSITY, THE EARTH & OUR HEALTH

*Biological diversity*, often shortened to **biodiversity**, is a term used to describe the vast variety of life on Earth. It refers to the magnitude of plants, animals, bacteria, and fungi that exist on our planet.[2] As you may recall, scientists estimate that there are at least 8.7 million species on the planet, encompassing all of its living creatures, plants, and microscopic organisms.

We primarily think of plants, animals, fungi, and bacteria as existing above ground or in the ocean . . . but in reality, *25 percent of the earth's biodiversity is found in the soil*.[3] Surprising, yes, but true! Soil is one of nature's most complex ecosystems: It contains a myriad of organisms that interact and contribute to the global cycles that make all life possible.

However, our soil is under threat, as so explicitly and thoroughly explained in the documentary *The Need to GROW*, which explores how we can feed the world and its growing population without destroying our farmable soil. According to Rob Herring, the producer, "We have about sixty years of viable soil left if we continue to deplete the soil at the going rate."[4] And because soil hosts a quarter of our planet's biodiversity, taking care of our soil is essential not only for food security and nutrition, but our health and wellness as well. So let's take a closer look at the soil: at what healthy soil means for us, and how getting your hands "dirty" can actually benefit your health.

## HOW SOIL & DIRT HELP OUR MICROBIOME

Healthy soil maintains a diverse community of organisms, both microscopic ones and ones you can see and feel, like earthworms and insects. Together, these organisms make up the *soil's microbiome*—what I like to call the "**soilbiome**" (I'm playing off the "soil is like the guts of the earth" idea here). Similar to how the health of your gut determines your overall health, the health of the soil determines the health of the plants that grow in it. The diversity of our soil affects the nutritional value of our fruits and vegetables—and that, in turn, affects the composition of our gut microbiome. And there's so much more to explain, so stick with me . . .

You've already heard about how microbial diversity among human beings is decreasing, and how, because of that, we have more gut issues than ever before. In the last century alone (and especially the last fifty years), we've seen a dramatic rise in gut-related problems. A study from the University of Gothenburg in Sweden found that for every ten adults in the world, four suffer from gastrointestinal disorders.[5] And trust me, that's not a coincidence. The increase in gut issues has a lot to do with the changes in the last fifty to a hundred years: pesticides, toxic environmental exposures, genetically modified crops, and more. What do all of these factors have in common? They all either affect or are affected by the health of our soil.

This is what I mean when I say, "*It's all interconnected.*" The soil impacts the plants; the plants affect your gut. Your gut also benefits from exposure to the microbes in the soil (I'll talk about this below). It's a multipronged, symbiotic relationship that can either help you live a long, full life with a healthy and happy gut and body . . . or wreak havoc on your gut and whole-body health, and eventually even endanger your life.

While we have limited immediate control over the amount of pesticides that are used worldwide, there are two things you can and should do now to benefit from the soil and the vast number of microbes it contains. First, become okay with getting dirty—getting out and getting your hands in the soil, because as I learned from my trip to the Hadza, the *soilbiome* helps diversify our gut microbiome. And second, vote with your dollars—by buying food that hasn't been grown with pesticides.

## GET DIRTY! WHY DIRT IS A GOOD THING

In truth, one of the easiest ways to increase microbial diversity in our guts is to expose ourselves to dirt and soil. (Remember how the Hadza didn't wash their hands, digging root vegetables out of the ground and eating them raw?) Inevitably, what gets on your hands gets to your gut as well. There, I said it: Get dirty!

In other words, get out into nature as much as you can. Don't be afraid of germs or getting dirty. Spend time in your garden. Run around your yard or a nearby park. Walk barefoot on the grass. Go for a long nature walk or hike. And stop scrubbing your *organic* produce with products designed to kill germs! Just rinse them with water. As long as a piece of produce is grown in pesticide-free soil, if a little dirt's left behind, all the more reason to eat it. All of this is good for your gut microbiome. It helps build diversity in the gut, which is reason enough on its own. But it also increases resilience in your body, making you more germ-proof than you may believe.[6]

Healthy exposure to environmental elements—getting our fingers dirty, spending time in nature, eating organic food straight from the earth—introduces *hormetic stressors* that make your gut microbiome more robust and your immune system more resilient. **Hormetic stress** is stress that challenges the body in a *good way*, like taking a cold shower or doing a *high-intensity interval training* (HIIT) workout. It forces the body to adapt by improving things like your metabolism and immune response. Adding weekly exposure to dirt and nature is a good "stress" *and* is stress-relieving for your whole body (as one study found, just 20 minutes outdoors can lower your levels of the stress hormone cortisol[7]). ***This is an important missing link in most people's gut-healing plans.***

I understand this might be a hard pill to swallow, especially if you're someone who values cleanliness or grew up in a household where dirt was demonized. But this kind of environmental exposure improves the diversity of your microbiome, and it will do so as a powerful adjunct to (or even better than) any gut-healing products you may try. Does that mean you can just get out in nature, maybe take up gardening, and ignore all the other gut-healing advice in this book? No, of course not! As a doctor and gut health guru, I have seen thousands of patients over more than two decades, and I know how critical a role diet, and often probiotic supplements (see more on these in chapter 7), play in healing the gut *and* the body. My point is that we *also* need healthy exposure to environmental elements—we need to get our fingers dirty, spend time in nature, and eat organic food straight from the earth when we can.

There's more. Not only is "getting dirty" actually a good thing for your gut, but the other side of the coin, overcleanliness—often viewed as a good thing—can actually be a bad one.

# THE PROBLEM WITH OVERCLEANLINESS

We've long been taught that dirt and germs are bad and that we should do everything in our power to get rid of them. So we wash, and we sanitize, destroying the microbes in our environment, on our food, and on our hands in the name of better health. Boy, do we have it backwards!

Contrary to popular belief, these collective "cleanliness" habits and our obsession with hygiene are actually working against us. We've been taught our entire lives that we should be washing our hands **constantly**, wiping down every surface we touch, and buying antibacterial and antimicrobial hand soaps and cleaning products. We are so focused on eliminating dirt and destroying germs that without realizing it, we have compromised our own gut, immune, and skin health.

Like antibiotics, sanitization was a major advance in medical treatment! Back in the latter half of the 1800s, Hungarian physician Ignaz Semmelweis[8] noted that pregnant women delivered by midwives were less likely to get potentially deadly postpartum infections because the midwives (unlike the doctors at the time) washed their hands between deliveries. He proposed obstetric doctors should wash their hands with a disinfectant solution between patients, but because this conflicted with the established scientific and medical opinions, it was rejected by the medical community. Years later, the germ theory of infection was confirmed by Louis Pasteur, and the rest his history. Of course, you wouldn't want your surgeon skipping the antibacterial soap. High levels of sanitation make absolute sense in the hospital setting, to prevent post-op infections. But in daily life, our obsession with strict sanitization is too much because of what it does to the skin and gut microbiomes.

The skin is the largest human organ, and it hosts a variety of bacteria and microbes that are crucial to our health. *Like the gut and the soil, the skin is home to millions of microorganisms.* When we go out in nature and get dirty, we are helping promote and maintain the diversity of the bacteria that live on the skin and in the gut. And unfortunately, behavioral practices like handwashing with antibacterial soaps or excessive use of antiseptic hand sanitizers *remove* these microorganisms, as well as the beneficial dirt, oil, and organic material that help form a healthy barrier on and maintain the homeostasis of the skin. Whereas plain soap binds to dirt and organic material while leaving the native skin microbiome undisturbed, antibacterial soaps are formulated to kill bacteria on our skin without discriminating between the good and the bad. Using these harsh products on your hands affects the microbiome on your skin surface and, if used too frequently, can break down the skin barrier. This can weaken your immunity, but it can also impact your gut flora, as several studies have shown.[9]

The ingredients in antibacterial products have come under fire in recent years because of the effect they have on gut health and our microbiota. In particular, **triclosan**—the active ingredient in antibacterial hand soap—has been shown to worsen colonic inflammation and alter the composition of our gut microbiome.[10] Triclosan is used in more than two thousand consumer products, including hand soap, toothpaste, mouthwash, clothes, kitchenware, and even toys. It's also been found in drinking water, and it can reach significant concentrations in the body. According to data from the National Health and Nutrition Examination, triclosan was detected in approximately 75 percent of the urine samples of individuals tested in the United States.[11]

In a similar vein, a 2018 study conducted in Madagascar found that antibacterial products impact the structure of microbial communities on the skin and have a lasting negative impact on skin microbes.[12] This suggests that removing beneficial bacteria and oils from our skin leads to a reduction in overall microbial diversity, which could thereby impair our immune system and skin barrier function.

As I've explained, favorable bacteria in your gut control the way that your immune system works and help keep your immune response in balance. In fact, certain bacterial strains, like *Lactobacillus rhamnosus*, trigger T-cells to mature into **T-regulatory cells**, which do as their name implies—they help "regulate" the immune system, keeping it from becoming overactive and causing damage to body tissues or, worse, leading to chronic disease.[13] And as you know from chapter 2, your skin—the largest organ in your body—is particularly susceptible to immune dysregulation.

## The Pandemic: A Microbial Diversity Killer

Speaking of bacteria-quashing global trends, the COVID-19 pandemic didn't do us any favors when it comes to microbial diversity. When the virus first came into the picture, scientists didn't know much about it. And because of that, people panicked, and most everyone erred on the side of oversanitization—namely, we over-used antibacterial and antimicrobial soaps, hand sanitizers, and cleaning wipes to disinfect ourselves and everything around us.

At the beginning, it made sense that we doubled down on san-itization, since we didn't know how the virus spreads, and no vac-cines or medical treatments were available to make it less deadly. That was worthwhile . . . but just like taking antibiotics, it came with a cost.

What we failed to recognize at the time was the impact this could have on our bodies and, most importantly, on our gut microbes. Studies done in 2020 revealed that exposure to house-hold disinfectants was associated with significant and detrimental changes in the composition and function of the intestinal flora, spe-cifically resulting in dysbiosis.[14] One of those studies highlighted emerging links between household cleaning products and antibi-otic resistance that might involve the gut microbiome.

Looking for a way to offset the negative impacts on gut micro-bial diversity of using lots of disinfectant during the early days of the pandemic? The researchers in the study recommended eating fermented foods in the hope of reversing dysbiosis—something I completely agree with based on my own research. (See more on the role of fermented foods in addressing gut imbalances in chap-ters 3 and 7.)

While antibacterial, antiseptic, and antimicrobial products can make us feel squeaky clean, they're actually detrimental to the body. Again, I'm not saying *never* wash your hands. Handwashing is a key way of preventing the spread of infec-tions. What I'm saying is ***don't overwash, don't oversanitize,*** and ***don't overclean*** to the point that you are disrupting the natural microbiome meant to diversify and protect us. Using regular hand soap (not antibacterial) and washing your hands thoroughly (front, back, and between the fingers) for the amount of time it takes to sing "Happy Birthday" is sufficient.

Exposure to dirt and the microbes within it is, as we've discussed, important in part because they are hormetic stressors that make your body stronger and more resistant to infection. But not all stressors are good, and there's a big environmental stressor that most people don't think about on a daily basis—pesticides.

## WHY PESTICIDES ARE BAD FOR YOUR GUT

At some point in your life, you were probably told by someone—a doctor, a health-conscious friend, a dietitian, or maybe even a farmer—that you should be buying organic food. You may have taken their suggestion, or you may have shaken it off, thinking you've made it this far eating nonorganic and nothing bad has happened. Why change now? I can't tell you how many times patients have questioned me, saying they are already healthy eaters. Why would buying organic make a difference? Well, I'm here to tell you there are **1 to 5.6 billion reasons why.** That's the amount in pounds of pesticides that are used on produce in the United States and worldwide, respectively.[15]

*In the US and globally, the agricultural industry is one of the two biggest current threats to biodiversity, in our gut and on our planet.* (The other is the healthcare industry and its overprescribing of antibiotics, as discussed in the previous chapter.) And pesticides are the primary reason.

Nonorganic produce is grown with loads of pesticides. As you may already know, the purpose of pesticides is to repel unwanted pests, like insects, rodents, weeds, and fungi, while produce is being grown and harvested. On the surface, this sounds like a good thing: Fewer pests means more produce available for harvest. However, these chemicals have been shown to have harmful effects on humans. In fact, pesticide exposure has been linked to an increased risk of developing numerous conditions, from cancer[16] to cognitive dysfunction[17] to Parkinson's disease[18] to cardiovascular disease[19] and even reduced fertility.[20] Studies have also found that children, whose brains and bodies are still developing, are especially susceptible to neurological damage caused by pesticide exposure.[21]

As if that wasn't bad enough, the pesticides and other chemicals used to grow conventional produce can cause dysbiosis that wreaks havoc on your gut health. The evidence is clear: Exposure to toxic environmental agents, like pesticides, can cause problems in your gut microbiome. And this is *in addition to* the harm they are causing to our gut health by destroying the biodiversity in our soil.

A study published in 2020 found that "environmentally induced perturbation in the gut microbiome is strongly associated with human disease risk."[22] To put it another way, toxic environmental chemicals have a detrimental effect on the gut microbiome, which then leads, as we've seen, to diseases associated with dysbiosis and leaky gut. These diseases include inflammatory bowel disease (IBD), obesity, diabetes, allergic conditions, skin rashes, cardiovascular disease, fatty liver, colorectal cancer, neurological disorders, and more. Most commonly, environmental toxins like pesticides can overwhelm your liver detox enzymes as well as lead to leaky gut.

## The US government does little to keep us safe from pesticides, despite the growing body of evidence that shows their harmful effects.

The US Environmental Protection Agency (EPA) does have limits on the amount of pesticides that can be used in commercial farming. But keep in mind, they're weighing the health risks (what happens to us) versus the reward (the money that commercial farms make and pay taxes on), so let's just say our best interests aren't exactly aligned with theirs.

### Glyphosate: The World's Worst Herbicide

No pesticide is "good" or beneficial to our health—not exactly shocking news, given that they're made of synthetic chemicals—but one of the most harmful is **glyphosate**, a widely popular herbicide used to kill weeds and unwanted grasses. If you look up the patent for glyphosate, you will find that it is registered as an *antimicrobial agent*, something that kills bacteria. But its primary purpose, for the purposes of the agriculture industry, is as a *chelating agent*, meaning it binds minerals, and thus starves weeds of the nutrients they need to live. Certain genetically modified crops have been designed to resist glyphosate (for example, Roundup Ready® corn and soy), which means that, when sprayed with glyphosate-containing pesticides, they survive while the weeds are destroyed.

However, they're still subject to glyphosate's mineral chelating action. As a result, the food you eat that has been sprayed with glyphosate is lower in nutrition than if it had been grown organically.

The most common crops genetically modified to be glyphosate-resistant are soy and corn. About 95 percent of these crops grown in the US are GMO, and it's estimated that farmers spray these crops with up to six times the amount of pesticide they would normally use, partly because weeds are becoming more resistant, requiring more and more pesticide to kill them off. (Remember how I talked about antibiotic resistance? Same idea here.) But other non-GMO crops, like wheat, are also sprayed with glyphosate, in order to mature it for harvest; as a result, non-organic wheat becomes contaminated with it. Wonder what all this glyphosate is doing to the soil? Well, one study showed that glyphosate disrupts the soil microbiome, destroying soil biodiversity and fertility.[23]

More importantly, *when glyphosate gets into the gut, it does the same thing: It binds minerals, starving your gut microbiome of necessary nutrients*. As a result, it can kill off good bacteria and lead to an overgrowth of pathogens in the gut—an imbalance in your gut flora, or dysbiosis—which then causes the gut lining to break down, leading to leaky gut and inflammation, which fuels the fires of chronic disease in the body.

Unfortunately, glyphosate is the most used herbicide in human history. Since 1974, 18.9 billion pounds of glyphosate have been sprayed worldwide. Take a second to fathom that number. **18.9 BILLION POUNDS!**[24] A Boeing 747 airplane weighs 404,600 pounds—so imagine 46,712 of those. Imagine 1,260,000 of the largest elephants in the world. That's how much glyphosate we're talking about here.

## A Public Health Crisis

Glyphosate exposure has been linked to increased risk of cancer, endocrine disruption, celiac disease, autism, and, you guessed it, leaky gut syndrome.[25] In 2015, glyphosate was reclassified as "probably carcinogenic" by the International Agency for Research on Cancer. Since then, many countries have limited or banned the use of glyphosate, including (at the time of publication) Bahrain, Belgium, Bermuda, Colombia, El Salvador, France, Kuwait, Netherlands, Oman, Qatar, Saudi Arabia, Sri Lanka, and United Arab Emirates.[26] Austria, Czech Republic, Denmark, France, Italy, Malawi, St. Vincent and the Grenadines, Thailand, and Vietnam have legislation limiting how much glyphosate can be used, most of which comes in the form of "partial bans," meaning glyphosate is being phased out of products but can still be used if there are no viable alternatives to the herbicide.[27]

At present, the US has **no ban** on glyphosate, despite the many pleas from human rights groups and concerned citizens. Based on the most recent available data, from 2016, the US used *287 million pounds* of glyphosate, up from 13.9 million pounds in 1992.[28] Of that 287 million, the Midwest alone accounted for an estimated 188.7 million pounds of glyphosate sprayed on crops, or about 65 percent of the nation's usage. When you consider that many of our most-consumed crops, like corn, wheat, and soy, are grown in Midwestern states, it's easy to see why scientists and consumers alike are concerned.[29] (Also, given glyphosate's impact on gut health, and gut health's impact on weight, it may be no surprise that when looking at historical CDC data, the obesity epidemic largely began in the Midwest.[30, 31]) Glyphosate use is an urgent issue for public health, and yet, our government is in no rush to ban glyphosate or any other pesticides.

Given how closely your health and disease risk is tied to your gut health (and the health of your gut microbe ecosystem), it's safe to say that avoiding pesticides is a smart decision for your overall well-being and longevity.

## HOW DO YOU PROTECT YOUR BIODIVERSITY?

At this point, I imagine you have many questions. *I'm just one person—what can I do about soil biodiversity? Is it even possible to heal my gut, given widespread pesticide use?* The answer is yes! And my GutSMART Protocol will teach you how to improve your gut health, feel great again, and even lose weight in the process. But there are plenty of additional steps you can take to increase your microbial diversity and, by proxy, begin to heal your gut.

Here are five changes I recommend making immediately to improve your gut health while having a positive impact on soil biodiversity:

1. ***Avoid excessive use of antiseptics, antimicrobials, and antibacterials.***

   I know how tempting it is to wash all of your food, disinfect all surfaces, and use hand sanitizer every time you touch something, but in doing so, you're messing with your skin microbiome and protective oils, and you're missing out on all the benefits that soil and environmental exposure has to offer, including the hormetic stress that allows your immune system to be in optimal shape.

   <u>To be clear</u>: I'm not saying you should put your hand on a subway pole and lick it. And I'm not saying you shouldn't wash your hands after using the restroom or before preparing food. Rather, I'm advising you to cut back on excessive use of hand sanitizers that can wipe out your skin microbiome and to cut out antibacterial and antimicrobial products; instead, wash your hands with regular soap.

2. ***Buy organic (if you can).***

   When you buy organic, you're not only supporting farmers who are helping to revive the biodiversity of our soil, but you're choosing to eat in a way that nurtures the health of your gut and body. As explained in the previous chapter, organic produce is richer in antioxidants, vitamins, and minerals than nonorganic produce. But the most important reason to buy organic is that it decreases your exposure to pesticides.

3. ***Follow the Dirty Dozen and Clean Fifteen lists.***

   I can't say it enough: In the interest of protecting your gut microbiome and gut lining, it's crucial that you find ways to minimize your pesticide exposure. If buying only organic produce isn't doable but you can afford to make a few swaps, I urge you to commit to buying produce according to the Environmental Working Group's "Dirty Dozen" and "Clean Fifteen" lists.

   The "Dirty Dozen," put together on a yearly basis, is a list of the fruits and vegetables contaminated with the highest levels of pesticides. These are the fruits and veggies you ideally ***always*** want to buy organic. The "Clean Fifteen" are the fruits and veggies that tend to have lowest levels of pesticide residue. These are the ones that you can feel safer buying conventional if you cannot find or afford to buy them organic.

To help you, I've included the lists for 2022 on pages 96 and 97. In truth, these lists don't change too significantly year to year, so regardless of when you're reading this, you can bet they are pretty close to the current recommendations. And you can always find the most up-to-date recommendations at EWG.org.

4. *Start your own organic garden at home.*

One positive outcome of the stay-at-home orders put in place during the COVID-19 pandemic? People started gardening! There's no time like the present to start your own vegetable garden at home. Not only is growing your own food a sustainable and potentially cost-saving choice, but if you grow your food in organic soil, you can drastically cut down on your pesticide exposure and thus help protect your gut from harm. Not to mention, it's another way to get dirty and expose yourself to the very important microbiome found in the soil.

5. *Find a farmer's market and do your produce shopping there.*

Reduce your pesticide exposure and the consequent harm to your gut by shopping at local farmer's markets. Even when using pesticides, smaller farms tend to use dramatically less than large-scale farms. And most farmer's markets have multiple vendors that are pesticide-free, even if they don't carry the organic label. Plus, by buying from farmer's markets, you'll support local farmers and get food closer to its source, which reduces its overall carbon footprint and ensures its freshness.

According to the USDA, there are over 8,600 farmer's markets in the US registered in their Farmers Market Directory, spread across all fifty states.[32] How easily you can access a farmer's market will depend on where you live, of course, but thanks to the internet, it's never been easier to find them. LocalHarvest.org has a Farmers Market Finder Tool you can use; just Google "local harvest farmers market finder" and type in your city and state.[33]

How you spend your money matters, so do it in ways that support what you believe in. By shopping organic and/or local when possible and avoiding mass-produced agriculture that has been sprayed with pesticides, you're voting with your wallet for a healthier world. Together, we have more power than you

# EWG - DIRTY DOZEN

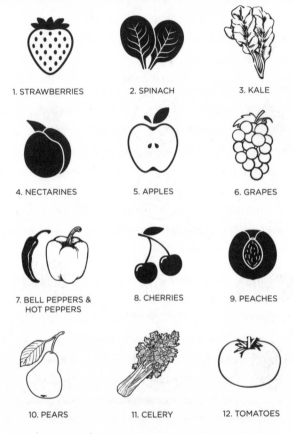

1. STRAWBERRIES   2. SPINACH   3. KALE

4. NECTARINES   5. APPLES   6. GRAPES

7. BELL PEPPERS & HOT PEPPERS   8. CHERRIES   9. PEACHES

10. PEARS   11. CELERY   12. TOMATOES

Copyright © Environmental Working Group, www.ewg.org. Reproduced with permission.

## More Ways to Support Your Local Farmer

There are many farms now that also deliver locally within their region to minimize their carbon footprint, and you can often order directly from them. Many of them also offer community-supported agriculture (CSA) shares, where they provide a box full of the freshest and most available seasonal produce on a weekly basis. You can find local CSAs by checking online or signing up for a community newsletter.

# EWG - CLEAN FIFTEEN

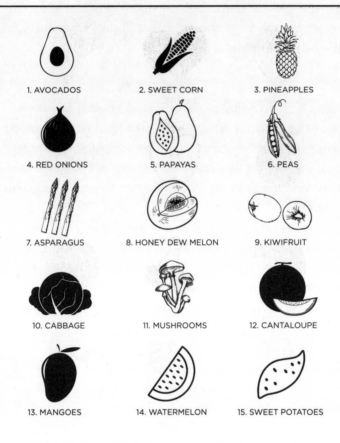

1. AVOCADOS     2. SWEET CORN     3. PINEAPPLES

4. RED ONIONS     5. PAPAYAS     6. PEAS

7. ASPARAGUS     8. HONEY DEW MELON     9. KIWIFRUIT

10. CABBAGE     11. MUSHROOMS     12. CANTALOUPE

13. MANGOES     14. WATERMELON     15. SWEET POTATOES

think to change policy. Look at all the countries that have banned glyphosate. Large corporations that disregard human health in the name of profits have no place in the future vision for humanity. Our voices (and pockets) united are more powerful than we give them credit for.

As we close this chapter, remember the words of Dr. Zach Bush: "Our gut microbiome is a direct extension of the nature that we touch." We are all interconnected. We both touch and are touched by the world around us. And societal changes that will have a positive impact on our collective health start with you. The small steps you take today to better your health will also better the health of the soil and the planet. Together, we can reverse the scourge of chronic disease that is plaguing the entire planet by first healing our guts. When we heal ourselves, we also help heal those around us by being examples of healthier living. We need to focus on what's truly important for our well-being—individually, together in community, and for the planet as a whole.

> "Our species is currently challenged with whether or not we will respect the infinite complexity within Nature's microscopic ecosystems. The influence of the micro-ecosystems cascades upwards into the macro-ecosystems, resulting in either chronic illness or sustained wellness, whether in people or an agricultural landscape.
>
> Do we want our farms to be abundant, productive, and resilient? Focus on the microbes. Do we want our bodies to have abundant energy, mental clarity, and physical resilience? Focus on the microbes."
>
> *—Rob Herring*

I invite you to do your part; start with at least one of the steps above, and become part of the movement by signing up for my newsletter at **HappyGutLife.com** to stay up to date with the latest.

## Takeaways

You did it! Another chapter down, and next, you get to begin your gut-healing journey by taking the GutSMART Quiz.

Before you move on, however, stop for a moment here to reflect on the highlights on the environmental impacts on your gut from this chapter:

1.  Your gut is connected to the environment around you—what happens in the outside world affects your inside world.

2.  We can't control the outside world, but we can control the choices we make as individuals that affect our health.

3.  Exposure to dirt, soil, and nature is extremely beneficial for the gut and, by proxy, your immune system. Don't be afraid to get your hands dirty and embrace the microbiome of the soil.

4.  Speaking of hands . . . stop oversanitizing. Hand sanitizers and antibacterial soaps deprive your skin of the oils and beneficial flora that protect the skin barrier. Instead, use regular soap to wash your hands.

5.  Conventional produce is loaded with pesticides, and these pesticides can disrupt the gut microbiome and cause leaky gut. Avoid pesticide-ridden produce by eating all organic if possible—or, at minimum, sticking to the "Clean Fifteen" for conventional produce and avoiding the "Dirty Dozen."

6.  Glyphosate is one of the most commonly used pesticides worldwide. It's best to avoid crops sprayed with it, not only because they are less nutritious due to glyphosate's chelating properties, but also because it can disrupt your gut microbiome by acting like an antimicrobial in your gut.

7.  If buying organic is too expensive, a second-best option is to buy locally, from farmer's markets. Smaller farmers tend to use fewer pesticides.

8.  Be conscious of what you spend your money on. As an individual, it's easy to feel like you can't make much of a difference in the realm of environmental awareness and sustainability, but you hold more power than you think. Purchasing patterns have power, and can make the difference between a local organic farm staying in business or a commercial farm forgoing pesticides. As part of a larger movement, *you, me, and—together—we* can make a really big difference in how food is grown and distributed both locally and globally.

# PART II

## GET GUTSMART!

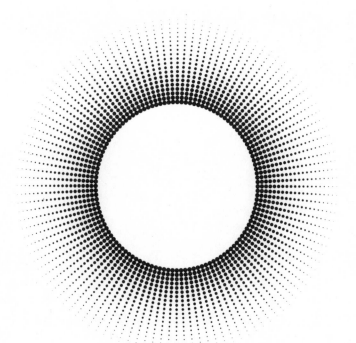

# Chapter 6

# THE GUTSMART QUIZ

> *"All the diets, plans, and protocols will be meaningless until you understand how they apply to you as an individual."*
>
> —Sarah Kay Hoffman (@agutsygirl)

**Have you ever noticed how easily you can get drawn into spending** five minutes taking a quiz to find out what medieval person, Disney character, or superhero you are most like? LOL. We love getting a new viewpoint on ourselves. The GutSMART Quiz won't tell you whether you are a princess or warrior, but it will help you gain a new perspective on the state of your health. It will tell you what level of gut impairment you have that may be holding you back from fully healing not just your gut, but the rest of your body as well. And it'll only take you a couple of minutes to complete.

Before we dive into the quiz itself, however, let's take a step back and put it into context.

# HOW THE GUTSMART QUIZ FITS INTO THE 14-DAY GUTSMART PROTOCOL

Taking the GutSMART Quiz is the first step before starting the 14-Day GutSMART Protocol. While there are a lot of factors affecting gut health, as explained in the previous chapters, the biggest one, and the one you have the most control over, is your diet. The quiz tells you which food category will best support your gut-healing journey. Based on your category—reflecting your level of gut dysfunction—you will tailor your diet to a personalized food list (see chapter 7). You can follow that category's meal plans or create your own (the recipes in chapter 9 can help!) to heal your gut and optimize your overall health and well-being in as little as fourteen days.

While there are only three categories in the protocol—Mild, Moderate, and Severe—your GutSMART Quiz score is unique to you and will most likely differ both from other readers and, most importantly, from your own *over time*. The ultimate goal as you follow the 14-Day GutSMART Protocol is to improve your score and feel the best you've felt in months (or even years!).

I want to make the process as simple as possible for you, so here's what to do:

1. Take the GutSMART Quiz and calculate your GutSMART Score.

2. Follow the GutSMART Protocol (chapter 7) for 14 days (two weeks).

3. Take the GutSMART Quiz again, see where you are, and re-evaluate.

4. Repeat the GutSMART 14-day Protocol based on your new score.

5. Repeat until you reach your lowest score possible and love how you feel.

The purpose of the GutSMART Quiz is twofold: (1) to determine which foods you *can* and *cannot* eat based on your score category, and (2) to gauge your progress—where you started versus where you are now. It's both an assessment tool and a progress-recording tool. Over the years, I've noticed that patients often don't realize how much progress they've made until I show it to them by pointing out specific improvements. By revealing your progress over time through scores you can compare, the quiz will make it easier to see how far you've come, and motivate you to keep going.

Here's an example of how the process might look: You start with a GutSMART Score in the Severe category, and after fourteen days, you've gone from Severe to Moderate; now, you can try eating some of the foods on the Moderate list and see how you feel. You do the Moderate plan for fourteen days, take the quiz again, and see if your gut has improved even more.

The GutSMART Protocol is designed to be repeated as needed—and to make eating for your gut type less stressful than ever before. I've seen patients go from Severe to Mild and then from Mild to feeling normal, with zero complaints, in just two to three months! But don't worry if this isn't you or you get stuck; I've got more tools to share with you, starting with Part IV, "Turbocharging Your Results," and more advice and resources, in "What's Next?—Living the GutSMART Life" and in the Appendix. I've got you covered no matter what!

## HOW TO TAKE THE GUTSMART QUIZ

The quiz is divided into sections that ask about groups of symptoms you may be experiencing solely in your gut, in your whole body, or both. Next to each symptom, you will find two columns. The first column asks for you to identify the *frequency* of your symptoms on a scale of 1 (never) to 5 (frequent). Answer as honestly and realistically as you can, choosing the number that best represents how often you experience each symptom *on average*. The second column asks you to identify the *severity* of your symptoms, also on a scale of 1 (not present) to 5 (severe). Try to answer based on what is most common when the symptoms occur.

This is followed by a series of additional questions that ask you to classify the frequency of use for various medications as well as indicate any recent weight gain. Again, be as honest as possible. This is for your benefit. The more accurately you answer the questions in this quiz, the more precise your score will be, which will help you get the most out of the GutSMART Protocol.

I ask about a lot of different symptoms to cover as wide a gut-related territory as possible (remember from chapter 2 that gut-related symptoms don't just happen in the gut!). That means the GutSMART Quiz is a bit longer than most health quizzes you may encounter, but by collecting more "data" about you, it allows us to be as accurate as possible. It also means that if you are unsure about how to rate the frequency or severity of a particular symptom, it's not going to affect your total score all that much. The quiz is designed to allow you to skip one to three questions if you're stumped and still get you in the right ballpark.

A final note before we start: Knowing yourself, try to provide the answer for each question that best characterizes what generally happens at your baseline, meaning outside of unusual circumstances (like postpartum or perimenstrual mood swings or during an acute infection you might have had right before you took the quiz), unless the related symptoms have become persistent, tend to happen on a regular basis, or come up more often than not.

Ready? Now let's get to it!

# THE GUTSMART QUIZ

Here's your scoring guide:

**For Symptom Frequency:**

1—Never

2—Rarely (less than 14 days total per year)

3—Occasionally (at least a few days or less each month, totaling no more than 4 weeks per year)

4—Regularly (3-15 days per month)

5—Frequently (daily or >15 days per month)

**For Symptom Severity:**

1—Not present

2—Mild

3—Moderate

4—Mostly moderate, sometimes severe

5—Always severe

What if you experience a symptom that is occasionally mild and only rarely moderate? If you answer "occasionally" (3) for frequency and "mild" (2) for severity, the total is 5. However, if you decide to answer with the worst severity and list "moderate" (3) but happening only "rarely" (2), you still get a total of 5. As long as you're answering the frequency and severity scores in relationship to one another, you should still get the same final score.

**How *often* do you experience the following symptoms? (Column 1)**

**How *severe* are the symptoms you experience? (Column 2)**

| THE GUTSMART QUIZ | Frequency + | Severity = | Total |
|---|---|---|---|
| Acid reflux/Heartburn | | | |
| Indigestion/Upset stomach | | | |
| Nausea | | | |
| Vomiting | | | |
| Constipation | | | |
| Diarrhea | | | |
| Alternating loose/hard stools | | | |
| Blood in stool‡ | | | |
| Mucus in stool | | | |
| White coating on the tongue§ | | | |
| Brown or yellow tongue coating | | | |
| Subtotal | | | |
| Bloating in between meals | | | |
| Bloating right after meals | | | |
| Food allergies | | | |
| Food sensitivities (see page 44) | | | |
| Sugar cravings | | | |
| Trouble with gluten/gluten intolerance* | | | |
| Lactose (dairy) intolerance** | | | |
| Overeating (inability to tell when full) | | | |

‡ If you see blood mixed with your stool, please seek the care and advice of a qualified healthcare professional for a diagnosis and treatment plan.

§ How to check if you have a coating on your tongue: (1) Get into the habit of looking at your tongue in the mirror every morning when you wake up, before brushing your teeth or drinking any fluids. (2) Check for a whitish, brownish, or yellowish film (could be subtle or thick like yogurt) at the base of the tongue (the part farthest away from your front teeth) daily for at least seven days. (3) If present every day, choose "5" for frequency. (4) Choose a severity, from 1 = barely visible to 5 = thick like a layer of yogurt on the tongue.

* When you have "trouble with gluten" or gluten intolerance, you may experience any of the following symptoms when you eat gluten-containing grains: feeling bloated after a meal, retaining water/puffy face, getting joint swelling or pain, or developing loose stools/diarrhea immediately or within a day or two.

** Lactose intolerance is most often characterized by bloating, abdominal pain, gas/flatulence, and diarrhea after eating dairy (lactose-containing) foods.

| THE GUTSMART QUIZ | Frequency + | Severity = | Total |
|---|---|---|---|
| Eating in a rush (inhaling your food) | | | |
| Subtotal | | | |
| Skin rashes (hives, eczema, rosacea, psoriasis) | | | |
| Acne | | | |
| Yeast infections | | | |
| Subtotal | | | |
| Tiredness or exhaustion (even with enough sleep) | | | |
| Dark circles under the eyes | | | |
| Bloodshot or red eyes | | | |
| Subtotal | | | |
| Seasonal allergies‡ | | | |
| Runny nose§ | | | |
| Sinus pressure or congestion | | | |
| Dry cough | | | |
| Asthma | | | |
| Subtotal | | | |
| Autoimmune disease (flare-ups) | | | |
| Hashimoto's hypothyroidism | | | |
| Subtotal | | | |
| Headaches | | | |
| Migraines | | | |
| Mental fog | | | |
| Mood swings | | | |
| Irregular/painful periods or hot flashes | | | |
| Subtotal | | | |
| Feeling stressed mentally | | | |
| Feeling stress in your gut* | | | |

‡ Think about whether you get seasonal (spring or fall) allergies every year, how frequently you suffer during allergy season, and how severe the symptoms are.
§ A runny nose can be a symptom of seasonal allergies, but it isn't always. It can also happen year-round, unrelated to allergy season, as a reaction to other airborne allergens, such as dust, dust mites, and animal dander.
* Feeling stress in your gut means that when you are stressed, you get a "knot" in your stomach or upset stomach, lose your appetite, eat emotionally, or even need to run to the bathroom with diarrhea.

| THE GUTSMART QUIZ | Frequency + | Severity = | Total |
|---|---|---|---|
| Worrying excessively | | | |
| Depression or low mood | | | |
| Anxiety or anxious mood | | | |
| Feeling consumed by work | | | |
| Subtotal | | | |
| **Symptoms Subtotal** (add up all subtotals) | | | |

You're almost there! Just a few more questions to go.

For the following questions, answer based on the *frequency* with which you have taken the medication or experienced the problem. This can be tricky when looking at antibiotics, because we want to capture use at any point in your lifetime (as they may have had long-term effects on the health of your gut microbiome). For example, if you took a lot of antibiotics as a child but not much as an adult, how would you rate it in terms of frequency? Your antibiotic use was very frequent years ago, but is rare now. In this case, you should give a score of 3, taking into account the high frequency in the past but the long amount of time that has passed since that frequent use. If you had taken a series of antibiotics more recently, then you would give it a higher score.

Remember that the test is designed to allow for some discrepancies in interpretation while still producing the same final result. So, don't get too caught up in the difference between answering 3 or 4 (for example) because the overall score is what matters most. As a reminder, here are the frequency scores again:

**For Symptom Frequency:**
1—Never
2—Rarely (less than 14 days total per year)
3—Occasionally (at least a few days each month or less, totaling no more than 4 weeks per year)
4—Regularly (3–15 days per month)
5—Frequently (daily or >15 days per month)

| | |
|---|---|
| How often have you taken tetracycline, doxycycline, or another antibiotic for acne for one month or longer?<br>*(If just one month or less a long time ago, answer 2. If multiple courses over 6 months or more, answer 5.)* | |
| How often have you taken an antibiotic at any point in your life, even just one course?<br>*(If just one course a long time ago, answer 2. If multiple courses in the last year, answer 5.)* | |
| How often have you taken over-the-counter pain medications, like ibuprofen (Advil) or acetaminophen (Tylenol), in the last year? | |
| Do you struggle with losing weight?<br>*(Answer based on how often you've dieted to lose weight in the last year.)* | |
| How frequently have you taken birth control pills in the last five years?<br>*(If not applicable to you, just answer 0.)* | |
| How much weight have you gained in the past five years? **Choose only one of the following**:<br><5 pounds (Score = 1)<br>5-10 pounds (Score = 2)<br>10-15 pounds (Score = 3)<br>15-20 pounds (Score = 4)<br>>20 pounds (Score = 5) | |
| **Questions Subtotal** | |

_____ + _____ = _____

Symptoms Subtotal    Questions Subtotal    Your GutSMART Score

# WHAT YOUR GUTSMART SCORE MEANS

Your GutSMART Score tells you your level of gut dysfunction—Mild, Moderate, or Severe:

| YOUR LEVEL | GutSMART Score |
|---|---|
| MILD | 25-150 |
| MODERATE | 151-350 |
| SEVERE | 351-450 |

- **MILD:** Your symptoms are of a mild nature and may occur only occasionally; however, they are significant enough to warrant following the 14-day protocol. Your goal is to have a lower score when you retake the quiz.
- **MODERATE:** This is the biggest category, and it means your symptoms are neither mild nor severe; they are in between. Your symptoms may be intermittent, happening more often than in the mild category, or they may be frequent but not severe. You will need to follow the 14-day protocol at least twice. Your goal is to move from Moderate to Mild when you retake the quiz.
- **SEVERE:** Your symptoms may be either acute or chronic in nature, but what distinguishes this category from the others is the degree of those symptoms. If you fall in this category, you have the most severe combination of symptoms. You will need to follow the 14-day protocol for at least three cycles. Your goal is to move from Severe to Moderate, then from Moderate to Mild, as you follow the protocol and retake the quiz at the end of each 14-day cycle.

Use the chart below to record your GutSMART Quiz score and the date you took the test. Then, use the chart again to mark your progress when you retake the quiz after completing each 14-Day GutSMART Protocol. Remember, retaking the test doesn't just allow you to track your progress. It also guides you as to which food list and meal plan to follow for optimum benefit during each two-week cycle, allowing you to stack together a personalized program for optimal gut-healing. Healing doesn't happen overnight—but I bet you'll be surprised by how much progress you can make in just two weeks!

| GUTSMART SCORE | YOUR LEVEL | DATE |
|---|---|---|
|  |  |  |
|  |  |  |
|  |  |  |
|  |  |  |
|  |  |  |
|  |  |  |

# GETTING GUTSMART

With your GutSMART Score in hand, I'm sure you're anxious to get started. But as tempting as it might be to jump to the recipes and meal plans right off the bat, I encourage you to first read the next chapter, because it's going to give you the final pieces of the puzzle you need to be successful. I'll show you how the GutSMART Protocol works and share with you important advice on how to navigate the meal plans and food lists, with some tips and tricks to help you further personalize the program according to your own needs.

I also want you to stop for a moment and reflect. Now that you've made it to this point in *The GutSMART Protocol*, you're smarter about how gut health affects the rest of your body and how the gut microbiome is a key collaborator in creating the wellness that you seek. Give yourself some love by reaching out with your arms and then wrapping them around yourself in a warm self-hug of success. You now know more about the gut than most of the world. Having this knowledge is the first step towards healing and living a healthy, happy gut life. So, you're already a winner in my eyes!

Now, let's roll up our sleeves together and get to work. You might want a notebook or sticky notes for the next chapter to jot down any important overarching concepts, ideas, or instructions you want to remember, so you can stick or tape them onto your fridge. You could even use your smartphone to take a picture or scan and print food lists and tape those to a prominent place in your home, somewhere you will see them every day while following the GutSMART Protocol. Or you can do as one young reader did with my last book: Carry it in your bag as a reference, highlighted and with multicolored sticky notes. (Just saying!)

But before you do that, I want you to do two things: (1) **write an affirmation**, and (2) **take and post a photo of yourself holding the affirmation**. Here's how: **Take a blank piece of paper. Grab a marker in your favorite color.** (By the way, did you know your favorite color represents how you view yourself? Just a little trivia for you!) Now write down this phrase:

## I'm GutSMART!! I CAN DO THIS!

Then, take a picture of yourself, post it on Instagram, and please tag me, **@drpedre**, as well as **@gut_smart**. Let's do this together! Let's create an allied community of GutSMART success stories!!

Finally, take that piece of paper and stick it on the wall in your bedroom—somewhere you'll see it first thing when you wake up every day. Why? Because it's going to give you the motivation you need for the next two weeks (and beyond) to wake up every day and follow the GutSMART Protocol—in spite of all the temptations, doubts, and setbacks that will inevitably try to get in the way of your success. I know you can do this. You wouldn't have picked up this book and read this far if you didn't believe you had it in you. And because you believe in yourself, I believe in you, too!

I'll see you in the next chapter, and don't forget to con-
nect with me on Instagram (**@drpedre**), where I post lots
of gut-centered inspirations to keep you going. I'm in it with
you 100 percent. Can I ask the same of you? Are you ready?
Are you committed? Are you in it 100 percent for yourself?
Take a *deep breath*. If the answer is yes, then *let's go!*

If the answer is no, then let me know what you need to
make it an *absolute yes*. You can even DM me on Instagram. Your mindset must be in the right place to be successful in any program you embark on, so if you're not ready yet, then skip to Part IV, "Turbocharging Your Results," and do the suggested exercises. They're not just useful for turbocharging your results. They can also help you overcome your internal resistance to change and put you in the best mindset possible to successfully complete the protocol.

I want you to feel great and energized in your body, have a happy belly and a clear mind, and be focused at work and ready to take on the world. **Let's get GutSMART!**

# Chapter 7

# THE 14-DAY GUTSMART PROTOCOL

> *"Let food be thy medicine and medicine be thy food."*
>
> —Hippocrates

**Now that you have your GutSMART Score, let's talk about how to** use it. In short, the GutSMART Protocol is a 14-day plan you will follow based on your score.

When it comes to eating right for your gut, there's no one-size-fits-all approach that works for everyone. That's why taking the GutSMART Quiz is so important. Knowing how to eat for your gut when it feels "out of whack" can be confusing. For example, some foods that are good for your gut *generally* may not be good or safe to eat if your gut dysfunction is currently severe. They may actually make your symptoms worse.

The GutSMART Quiz puts you into a category that tells you what foods are best for your gut based on your current level of gut impairment, and which ones to avoid. However, before we get into that in-depth, I want to start with a bird's-eye view. First, I'll share the general principles that apply to everyone, regardless of your GutSMART Score. Then, we'll get personal by showing you what foods are allowed for the different levels—Mild, Moderate, and Severe—and how to personalize your 14-day GutSMART Protocol for optimal gut healing.

# WHAT TO EAT FOR OPTIMAL GUT HEALTH

Whenever I tell my patients they will need to change their diet to improve their gut health, their first question is, "So *what* can I eat?" It can feel daunting to think about sacrificing some foods that you really enjoy—even if they make your gut or body sick.

When it comes to eating, we tend to follow our emotions more than our logic. And our emotions often override what we truly know deep down inside—that a certain food or beverage is not right for us. So, one important piece of the protocol is to nurture that "inner knowing," or paying attention to how your body reacts to different foods or drinks—in other words, how they make you feel, physically and emotionally. This intuitive muscle will help you fine-tune a way of eating that honors your individuality. (In the "Intuitive Eating" section towards the end of this chapter, I go into more detail about how to develop that inner sense around eating.)

With the help of nutritionists, an understanding of the power of a diet low in FODMAPs (see pages 44–45) to improve IBS-like symptoms, and my own clinical experience, I have put together a food list that is divided into three categories, each corresponding to a GutSMART Score: Mild, Moderate, and Severe. It is the most exhaustive food list I have ever seen anywhere, and is designed to tell you what you *can* eat, depending on your score, so you can make the *best choices* for yourself and your gut-healing journey.

The heart of the 14-Day GutSMART Protocol is these categorized lists of foods, because let's be realistic—very few people prepare every single meal they eat themselves. To be able to follow this protocol even while eating out or ordering in, an exhaustive food list was needed that addresses the individuality that results from varying levels of gut dysfunction.

There are also certain superfoods, like ginger and turmeric, that have an incredible, positive effect on the gut, and I've included these in the "Foods That Heal and Soothe the Gut" section below the food list.

But before we get to the GutSMART Food List, let's start at the macro level, with what's *generally* safe and healthy to eat for a healthy gut. (We'll break it down for each category when we get to the food list.) When embarking on any gut-healing protocol, it's important to focus on the vast amount of foods that will nurture the gut and help reverse the negative impact of months (or even years) of poor eating habits—not just what you have to avoid.

## What to *Enjoy* Eating

Organic, non-GMO vegetables,¥ ideally nonstarchy or low-starch varieties*

High-fiber, low-glycemic carbs

Healthy (omega-3) fats

Grass-fed ghee<sup>ʏ</sup>

Nuts, seeds¥

Berries, other low-sugar fruit¥

Fermented foods¥

Hypoallergenic proteins (pea, rice, chia, chickpea, and hemp)

Clean and lean proteins:

    Hormone-free, pasture-raised beef and lamb

    Free-range chicken and turkey

    Wild-caught cold-water fish (no farmed fish)

    Wild game (bison, Cornish hen, duck, elk, pheasant, venison, kangaroo, ostrich)

¥ These are not allowed equally in every category. See details in food lists below.

* These should replace high-glycemic carbs for Severe and Moderate scores.

ʏ Even if you have a dairy sensitivity, you should be fine eating **ghee**, or clarified butter, because it is devoid of dairy proteins, but avoid or limit its use if your dairy sensitivity is severe.

The foods you *can* eat encompass broad categories that research has shown benefit our health and well-being, but even a healthy food might be problematic for some individuals. For example, nuts are great sources of protein and omega-3 fatty acids, but if you have a nut allergy or sensitivity, you would obviously want to avoid them, regardless of their positive health effects. Another example is pea protein. The majority of people don't have an allergy or sensitivity to pea protein, making it one of the safest hypoallergenic protein options in vegan protein powders, but a small minority do and therefore should avoid it. So again, these are general guidelines. You should customize them to fit your individual circumstances, and of course, follow the specific recommendations under your GutSMART Score category.

# TOP FOOD & DRINK CATEGORIES
# TO AVOID OR LIMIT

Now a take a deep breath and let it out slowly with a sigh. Ahhh! I want to talk to you about a few big categories of foods (and beverages) that are harmful to the gut in a large portion of the world population. The top two categories of foods to avoid are **wheat/gluten** and **dairy**. Research has shown that gluten increases the likelihood of leaky gut, even in normal individuals with no underlying gut issues. And a majority of people (about 75 percent worldwide) either are lactose intolerant or suffer from hidden dairy sensitivities that make consuming dairy an attack on their gut.

When it comes to beverages, you probably won't be surprised that **alcohol** is *out* during the 14-Day GutSMART Protocol, and **coffee** is either out or markedly reduced. If you're serious about healing your gut, especially when you have Moderate or Severe dysfunction, then avoiding alcohol is a prerequisite. The amount of sugar in many alcoholic beverages, including mixed drinks and wine, messes with the balance of your gut flora. Many wines are overly acidic and can aggravate acid reflux. And beer is filled with yeast that can lead to auto-fermentation in the gut, leading to uncomfortable gas and bloating.

Why cut back on coffee when healing your gut? Four main reasons:

1. Coffee tends to be very acidic, increasing stomach acid production and aggravating acid reflux for many.

2. Coffee irritates the gut lining, which can lead to diarrhea or loose stools.

3. Coffee beans tend to be contaminated with mold, which is harmful to the gut.

4. Coffee disrupts restful deep sleep.

Now remember, we're talking macro level here. Once you get into the micro level in the food list, you'll see that as your gut dysfunction improves from Severe to Moderate to Mild, certain foods (and even certain alcohols) can be allowed back in. There is a light at the end of the protocol tunnel!

Here are the broad categories of foods and drinks you should avoid because they will make your gut sicker, leading to uncomfortable bloating, constipation, and/or diarrhea, and aggravate gut-related symptoms, while hindering your progress towards feeling great again.

## What to *Avoid* Eating & Drinking

Wheat/gluten

Raw cruciferous vegetables (kale, broccoli, cauliflower)

Lentils, beans[§]

GMO corn

GMO soy

Hydrogenated vegetable oils, trans fats

Select fruits[*]

Dairy, butter[£]

Farm-raised fish

Grain-raised meats

Nonorganic, factory-raised eggs

Coffee[¥]

Alcohol

Carbonated beverages/sparkling water[Y]

Processed or artificial sugars

---

[§]  If you are vegan or vegetarian and need to eat beans and lentils as a protein source, you can enjoy them as part of a gut-friendly diet when they are properly prepared (see page 135). However, if you are in the Severe category, limit them as much as possible as per the food list until you progress to the Moderate category.

[*]  See categorized foods below for more details.

[£]  See categorized foods below for more details. For example, grass-fed ghee is okay even in the Severe category, but butter is not.

ˣ Either cut out coffee altogether or limit it to one 8-ounce cup daily. For some people, coffee serves as a laxative, helping to prevent constipation; if that's you, then cut back, but don't cut it out completely.

ʸ Especially for the Moderate and Severe categories, sparkling water and carbonated beverages can increase uncomfortable bloating and gas. It's best to avoid them entirely or limit them.

# THE GUTSMART FOOD GUIDE

Now that you have a bird's-eye view on how to eat for your gut health, let's dive into the details. The chart below lists the foods that are safest for each GutSMART category—Mild, Moderate, and Severe. For example, if you tested Severe, then you should stick with the foods in the Severe column and avoid the others. It doesn't mean you have to eat all of the foods in your category. To avoid getting overwhelmed, think of this list more like a guide that you'll use when grocery shopping or eating out. Don't try to memorize it! It's here to provide direction on what you *can* eat, so that you keep in mind the huge variety of foods you have to choose from, regardless of your score. It's meant to keep you from feeling deprived.

## How to Use the Food List

· In the following chart, you'll find foods listed according to the category they best belong in. Some foods will have suggested quantities listed, sometimes with a less than (<) or greater than (>) sign. You should use Intuitive Eating (see below) to determine how much of each food works best for you. For example, if you're in the Mild category, you can have >1 cup broccoli, but you may find that, for you, 2 cups is *too much* and makes you feel bloated, and that you need to limit broccoli to 1 or 1½ cups.

- For foods you're not sure about, the best thing to do is listen to your gut. Test them in smaller quantities first, then increase as tolerated or as your GutSMART Quiz score improves.

- If a food appears in the Severe category but not in Moderate or Mild, that doesn't mean that you can't eat it if you score Moderate or Mild. The lists are additive. Those who score Mild can (and should!) eat across all categories, including Moderate and Severe. Moderates can eat foods in both the Moderate and Severe categories. Severes should limit themselves to *only* foods in the Severe category.

- When eating vegetables, the more severe your gut dysfunction is, the more cooked your vegetables should be in order to avoid uncomfortable bloating, gas, and abdominal pain.

  - *Severe*: Stick to cooked vegetables as much as possible. Cooking vegetables starts the process of breaking down their hard-to-digest plant cell wall components into usable nutrients before you eat them and reduces gut-harming anti-nutrients, which in turn eases digestion.

  - *Moderate*: Start with a mix of cooked and raw vegetables in up to a 2:1 ratio per meal, and then move closer to a 1:1 ratio as your gut dysfunction improves.

  - *Mild*: You can eat a mix of cooked and raw veggies in up to a 1:1 ratio per meal or consume all cooked or all raw veggies in one sitting, as in a large salad.

# THE GUTSMART FOOD LIST[‡]

| SEVERE | MODERATE | MILD |
|---|---|---|
| **VEGETABLES** | | |
| Artichoke hearts: 2 tablespoons | Asparagus, 1 spear | Artichoke |
| Bamboo shoots | Artichoke hearts, ¼ cup | Asparagus: 4 spears |
| Beet: 2 slices | Bok choy, yu choy, gai choy, 1 cup | Beet: 4 slices |
| Bell pepper | Butternut squash, ½ cup | Bok choy: 1½ cups |
| Broccoli: ½ cup | Broccoli, <1 cup | Broccoli: >1 cup |
| Broccoli rabe | Cabbage: red or green, >1 cup | Brussels sprouts: 6 |
| Cabbage, red or green: 1 cup | Cabbage, napa (Chinese cabbage), ¾ cup | Butternut squash: 1 cup |
| Cabbage, savoy: ½ cup | Cabbage: savoy, ¾ cup | Cabbage, savoy: 1 cup |
| Carrot | Celery: 1 stalk | Cauliflower |
| Celery: ⅓ stalk | Chili pepper: 2 tablespoons | Celery: >1 stalk |
| Celery root (celeriac) | Chinese celery | Chili peppers: ¼ cup |
| Chives | Fennel bulb, ½ cup | Fennel bulb: >1 cup chopped |
| Cucumber | Gai lan (aka Chinese broccoli) | Fennel fronds: >3 cups |
| Eggplant | Leek: ½ | Garlic |
| Endive | Parsnip | Hearts of palm |
| Escarole | Peas: ⅓ cup | Jicama |
| Fennel bulb: ¼ cup | Pea shoots (pea tips, leaves, tendrils) | Jerusalem artichoke (aka sunchoke) |
| Green beans: 10 | Potato, purple: <½ cup | Kohlrabi |
| Greens (arugula, collard, dandelion, lettuce, kale, mustard, spinach, chard, microgreens, beet, turnip, carrot leaves, radish greens) | Spinach, water spinach: >15 leaves | Leek |
| Olives | Sweet potato: ½ cup | Mushrooms |
| Peas: ¼ cup | | Onions, yellow, red, spring |
| Radicchio: 12 leaves | | Peas: ½ cup |
| Radish (daikon, French, watermelon) | | Potatoes, white, red; purple: >½ cup |
| Rutabaga | | Radicchio: >12 leaves |
| Scallion, green part | | Seaweeds/sea vegetables |
| Snow peas: 5 pods | | Snow peas: 10 pods |
| Sprouts (all types) | | Scallions |
| Squash (acorn, butternut, chayote, kabocha, pumpkin puree): ¼ cup | | Shallots |
| Sweet potato, ¼ cup | | Sugar snap peas |
| Watercress: 12 leaves | | Sweet potato: >½ cup |
| Zucchini, yellow squash: ¾ cup | | Tomatillo |
| | | Tomato |
| | | Tomato, paste, soup, sauce, juice |
| | | Tomato, sun-dried: 2 tablespoons |
| | | Turnip |
| | | Taro |
| | | Water chestnuts |
| | | Watercress: >12 leaves |
| | | Yam |
| | | Yucca |
| | | Zucchini, yellow squash: >¾ cup |

‡ I want to thank Monash University for creating an extensive *Low FODMAP Certified Foods Guide* and Dr. Allison Siebecker for her pioneering work in creating a multi-level *SIBO Specific Diet: Food Guide* for patients suffering from SIBO (small intestine bacterial overgrowth). Both served as an inspiration for creating this very detailed, tiered food list. If you have SIBO, please check out SIBOinfo.com. For a detailed Low FODMAP Diet, you can also download the Monash University FODMAP Diet App.

| SEVERE | MODERATE | MILD |
|---|---|---|
| **FRUIT** | | |
| Avocado: ¼ small | Avocado: ½ small/medium | Apple |
| Banana: fresh or dried | Cherries: 3 | Apricot, fresh or dried |
| Blueberries: <⅔ cup | Cranberries: 10 (2 | Avocado |
| Boysenberries: 10 |    tablespoons) | Blackberries: >50 |
| Carambola | Grapefruit: ½ | Blueberries: >⅔ cup |
| Camu camu | Longan: 10 (¼ cup) | Cherries: 6 |
| Currants: 1 tablespoon | Lychee: 5 (2 tablespoons) | Cranberries: 2 tablespoons |
| Dragon fruit | Melon, cantaloupe or | Custard apple‡ |
| Durian |    honeydew: <½ cup | Date, dried and soaked |
| Guava | Passion fruit | Fig, dried |
| Kiwifruit | Pear, Asian, peeled | Gooseberry |
| Kumquats | Pineapple, dried: 1 slice | Grapefruit: 1 |
| Lemon | Rambutan: <⅓ cup | Grapes |
| Lime | | Jackfruit |
| Longan: 5 | | Jam/jelly, homemade (no |
| Orange | |    pectin or sugar) |
| Papaya | | Mango§ |
| Passion fruit: ⅔ cup | | Melon, cantaloupe or |
| Pawpaw | |    honeydew: >½ cup |
| Pineapple | | Nectarine |
| Pomegranate: ¼ cup seeds | | Papaya, dried |
| Prickly pear | | Peach |
| Rambutan: 2 | | Pear |
| Raspberries: 10 | | Persimmon |
| Rhubarb | | Plantain |
| Strawberries: 10 | | Plum |
| Tangerine, tangelo | | Pomegranate: ½ cup seeds |
| | | Prunes |
| | | Raisins |
| | | Raspberries: >50 |
| | | Tamarillo§ |
| | | Watermelon |

‡ Also known as an "atis" in the Philippines, sugar apple, or sweet-sop.
§ May need to avoid if fructose-intolerant.

| SEVERE | MODERATE | MILD |
|--------|----------|------|
| **DAIRY / DAIRY SUBSTITUTES** | | |
| Almond milk, homemade<br>Cashew milk, homemade:<br>  1½ cups<br>Coconut milk, homemade<br>Coconut milk, commercial<br>  (without thickeners)<br>Ghee, <1 tablespoon<br>Hemp milk, commercial<br>  (without thickeners): 1½<br>  cups<br>Macadamia milk:<br>  homemade, 1½ cups<br>Rice milk, homemade: 1½<br>  cups | Butter, cultured, grass-fed<br>Cheese: hard, aged<br>  1 month or more,<br>  parmesan, Romano,<br>  yogurt cheese/labneh<br>Coconut milk yogurt,<br>  commercial: 1<br>  teaspoon–¼ cup<br>Flax milk, homemade: 1½<br>  cups<br>Ghee: <2 tablespoons<br>Kefir: 48-hour fermented<br>  homemade, goat, cow: 1<br>  teaspoon–¼ cup<br>Oat milk, commercial<br>  (without thickeners): 1½<br>  cups<br>Pili nut yogurt, commercial,<br>  1 teaspoon–¼ cup<br>Sour cream, 24-hour<br>  fermented homemade:<br>  2–3 tablespoons<br>Yogurt, 24-hour<br>  fermented homemade: 1<br>  teaspoon–¼ cup | Butter, grass-fed<br>Cheese: cream cheese,<br>  cottage cheese, dry<br>  curd cottage cheese,‡<br>  feta, goat cheese, fresh<br>  mozzarella, ricotta<br>Kefir, commercial, 48-hour<br>  fermented homemade,<br>  plain, goat<br>Milk, cow (A2)<br>Milk, sheep, goat, camel<br>Yogurt, plain, Greek, goat,<br>  sheep |

---

‡ I recommend Nancy's Organic Fermented Cottage Cheese.

| SEVERE | MODERATE | MILD |
|---|---|---|
| **GLUTEN-FREE GRAINS, FLOURS + STARCHES** | | |
| Almond flour: 2 tablespoons<br>Coconut flour<br>Plantain flour<br>Rice, white: ½ cup, cooked | Amaranth<br>Almond flour<br>Arrowroot (flour)<br>Baking powder (gluten-free)<br>Baking soda<br>Buckwheat<br>Buckwheat groats<br>Cornstarch<br>Hazelnut flour<br>Mesquite flour‡<br>Millet<br>Montina flour§<br>Nut flour/nut meal<br>Oats (gluten-free)<br>Pea flour<br>Potato flour, starch<br>Quinoa flour, whole<br>Quinoa flakes<br>Rice, brown, white: 1 cup<br>Rice bran<br>Sago (starch)<br>Sorghum flour<br>Tapioca starch (manioc, cassava, yucca)<br>Teff flour | Bean flours: garbanzo, fava, Romano<br>Flaxseed meal, golden, brown: 1 tablespoon<br>Gums: guar, xanthan*<br>Rice, wild rice, brown, white |
| **BEANS** | | |
| Adzuki beans, sprouted: ¼–½ cup<br>Sprouted mung beans, ¼–½ cup | Adzuki beans, sprouted: ¾ cup<br>Black: ½ cup<br>Lentils, green, red: ¼ cup<br>Lima, cooked ⅓ cup<br>Mung beans, sprouted: ¾ cup | Adzuki beans, sprouted: 1 cup<br>Chickpea (garbanzo), fava, broad, kidney, red<br>Lentils, brown, red, green: ½ cup<br>Lima: ½ cup<br>Mung beans, sprouted: 1 cup<br>Navy, white, haricot<br>Spilt peas |

‡ A little-known superfood from North America, mesquite flour (made from milled seeds) is gluten-free, rich in protein (17%), minerals, and the essential amino acid lysine. Don't let the sweet taste—a mix of cocoa, molasses, and hazelnut—fool you. Mesquite flour is low in sugar impact and high in fiber content. Great to use in gluten-free desserts!

§ Made from milled Indian ricegrass, Montina flour is gluten-free and can be mixed with other gluten-free flours to make gluten-free pizza dough.

* Neither guar gum nor xanthan gum are technically starches, but like starches, they are polysaccharides and act like starches in helping to thicken foods (up to eight times), like sauces, gravies, and nut milks. Beware that some people will react negatively to these gums with gas, bloating, and loose stools. If that's the case, then try to avoid them.

| SEVERE | MODERATE | MILD |
|---|---|---|
| **MEAT + FISH** | | |
| Anchovies<br>Bacon, uncured, preservative-free<br>Beef, grass-fed<br>Bison, grass-fed<br>Bone broth, homemade, meat or bone marrow (no cartilage)<br>Cornish hen<br>Duck<br>Fish, wild-caught<br>Ham, preservative-free<br>Lamb, grass-fed<br>Organ meats (from grass-fed animals)<br>Pork, hormone-free, antibiotic-free<br>Poultry, hormone-free, antibiotic-free<br>Quail<br>Sardines<br>Shellfish, wild-caught<br>Veal, grass-fed<br>Venison<br>Wild game (elk, bison, venison, pheasant, kangaroo, ostrich) | Eggs, chicken, duck, quail; pasture-raised, organic: soft-boiled, sunny-side up | Bone broth, homemade, bone/cartilage<br>Eggs, chicken, duck, quail; pasture-raised, organic: frittata, soft omelet, soft scrambled |

| SEVERE | MODERATE | MILD |
|---|---|---|
| **NUTS + SEEDS** | | |
| Almonds, sprouted: 10<br>Brazil nuts: 2<br>Carob/locust bean gum/<br>   carob gum<br>Hazelnuts: 10 (2<br>   tablespoons)<br>Hemp seeds: 1 teaspoon<br>Macadamia nuts: 20 (⅓<br>   cup)<br>Pecans: 10 (<¼ cup)<br>Pine nuts: 1 tablespoon<br>Pumpkin seeds, sprouted:<br>   2 tablespoons<br>Sesame seeds: 1<br>   tablespoon<br>Sunflower seeds, sprouted:<br>   2 tablespoons<br>Walnuts: 10 (<¼ cup) | Brazil nuts: 4<br>Chestnuts: 5–7<br>Cacao, powdered/raw,<br>   alkali-free<br>Coconut, shredded or<br>   flaked: ¼ cup<br>Hazelnuts: 20 (¼ cup)<br>Hemp seeds: ≤ 2 teaspoons<br>Pecans: 40 (<⅔ cup)<br>Pine nuts: ¼ cup<br>Poppy seeds: 1 teaspoon<br>Walnuts: <⅔ cup | Almonds, sprouted or dry-<br>   roasted: 20<br>Barùka nuts‡<br>Brazil nuts: 5–10<br>Cacao nibs<br>Caraway seeds<br>Cashews: ~20<br>Chia seeds<br>Coconut milk with<br>   thickeners (guar gum,<br>   tapioca starch)<br>Flaxseeds, ground: >1<br>   tablespoon<br>Hazelnuts: 80<br>Hemp seeds: ≤1 tablespoon<br>Pili nuts<br>Pine nuts: ½ cup<br>Pistachios<br>Poppy seeds: <1<br>   tablespoon<br>Poppy seeds, sprouted:<br>   <⅓ cup<br>Pumpkin seeds, sprouted:<br>   <⅔ cup<br>Sacha inchi<br>Seed flours<br>Sesame seeds: <⅔ cup<br>Sunflower seeds, sprouted<br>   or dry-roasted: <⅔ cup<br>Walnuts: <1 cup |
| **VEGETABLE PROTEINS** | | |
| Bee pollen<br>Blue-green algae<br>   (chlorella)<br>Chickpea protein<br>Pea protein: micronized§<br>Sacha inchi protein<br>Spirulina<br>Rice protein | Hemp protein<br>Pea protein, regular<br>Pumpkin seed protein<br>Vegetable protein blends<br>   (like quinoa/amaranth) | |

‡ One of my favorite brands is Barùkas, found at Barukas.com.
§ For example, the HAPPY GUT Cleanse Shake or Nourish protein powder meal replacement.

| SEVERE | MODERATE | MILD |
|---|---|---|
| **FATS + OILS** | | |
| Algae oil‡<br>Avocado oil<br>Coconut oil, extra virgin or refined<br>Cod liver oil<br>Fish oil<br>Ghee, grass-fed<br>Medium-chain triglyceride (MCT) oil<br>Macadamia oil<br>Olive oil, cold-pressed, extra virgin | Bacon fat, pasture-raised<br>Cacao butter<br>Coconut butter: 1 tablespoon<br>Coconut cream: 1 tablespoon<br>Coconut oil, unrefined<br>Duck fat<br>Polyunsaturated borage, flax, hemp, pumpkin seed, sacha inchi, walnut oil (cold only) | Coconut cream: >1 tablespoon<br>Garlic-infused olive oil<br>Polyunsaturated grapeseed, sesame, sunflower oil (for occasional cooking, frying, stir-frying) |
| **HERBS + SPICES** | | |
| Asafetida (hing)<br>Basil<br>Bay leaves<br>Cardamom<br>Cilantro<br>Cloves, ground<br>Coriander, ground<br>Cumin tea (not cooking spice)<br>Dill<br>Fennel seed<br>Makrut/thai lime leaves<br>Lemongrass<br>Oregano<br>Parsley<br>Pepper, black<br>Rosemary<br>Sage<br>Sea salt<br>Star anise<br>Tarragon<br>Thyme | Cinnamon, whole stick or ground<br>Chives<br>Cumin, ground: 1 teaspoon<br>Curry leaf<br>Curry powder: 1 teaspoon<br>Galangal<br>Ginger, fresh or dried<br>Mint<br>Nutmeg, ground<br>Paprika, sweet<br>Turmeric, fresh or dried | Chili flakes, dried<br>Cumin, ground: >1 teaspoon<br>Curry powder: >1 teaspoon<br>Garlic powder<br>Onion powder<br>Paprika, smoked |

‡ For example, Thrive Culinary Algae Oil.

| SEVERE | MODERATE | MILD |
|---|---|---|
| **CONDIMENTS** | | |
| Bragg's Liquid Aminos<br>Liquid coconut aminos<br>Dulse flakes<br>Fennel seeds (as a digestive and breath freshener)<br>Mayonnaise, homemade or commercial (with avocado oil)<br>Mustard, stone-ground<br>Nutritional yeast<br>Tamari<br>Vanilla beans<br>Vanilla flavoring (alcohol-free)<br>Vanilla powder | Vinegar, apple cider (organic), distilled‡ white, red wine, white wine<br>Mustard, Dijon<br>Pickles, relish (no sweetener or garlic)§<br>Tahini: 1 tablespoon | Barbecue sauce, gluten-free, unsweetened*<br>Horseradish<br>Hot sauce<br>Ketchup: organic, unsweetened**<br>Tahini: >1 tablespoon<br>Relish/chutney<br>Vinegar, balsamic, white balsamic<br>Wasabi, pure |
| **FERMENTS††** | | |
| | Beet kvass: 1–3 teaspoons<br>Brine-cured olives: 1–5 (<¼ cup)<br>Coconut water kefir, low-sugar (≤7 grams), <¼ cup/day<br>Fermented veggies<br>Kimchi brine, not spicy, raw, unpasteurized: 1 teaspoon<br>Miso, red: 1–3 teaspoons<br>Pickles, lacto-fermented: ½–1<br>Sauerkraut brine, raw, unpasteurized: 1 teaspoon<br>Water kefir: low-sugar (≤7 grams): <¼ cup/day | Beet kvass: >1 tablespoon (<¼ cup/day)<br>Brine-cured olives: ¼–½ cup<br>Coconut water kefir, low-sugar (≤7 grams), <½ cup/day<br>Kimchi, spicy: 2 tablespoons<br>Kombucha, low-sugar (≤7 grams): <½ cup/day<br>Miso, red: >1 tablespoon<br>Miso, white: 1–3 teaspoons<br>Pickles, lacto-fermented: 2–3<br>Sauerkraut: 1–2 tablespoons<br>Sauerkraut brine, raw, unpasteurized: 2 tablespoons<br>Water kefir, low-sugar (≤7 grams), <½ cup/day |

‡ Note that plain distilled vinegars are gluten-free even when made from gluten-containing grains. Gluten is removed during the distillation process, rendering the final product gluten-free. That said, if you have celiac disease, exercise caution when trying a distilled vinegar by testing a small amount first and making sure it doesn't cause a reaction.

§ See "Ferments" below for details.

* For example, Primal Kitchen Organic Unsweetened BBQ Sauce.

** For example, Primal Kitchen Organic Unsweetened Ketchup.

†† For all ferments in the Moderate category, start with a small amount and increase the quantity slowly. Watch out for added sugar in commercial brands. It's best to buy plain because they will have the least amount of added sugar.

| SEVERE | MODERATE | MILD |
|---|---|---|
| **BEVERAGES** | | |
| Aloe vera juice: ¼–½ cup/ day<br>Coconut water: ¼–½ cup<br>Nut milk, unsweetened, carrageenan-free (see Dairy/Dairy Substitutes)<br>Tea, black (weak), chamomile, dandelion, hibiscus, lemongrass, matcha, mint, nettle, oolong, rooibos/rooibos chai, rose hip<br>Water, filtered; reverse-osmosis (if possible) | Aloe vera juice: ≤1 cup/day<br>Carbonated beverages, no sugar<br>Coconut water<br>Seltzer: ≤1 cup/day<br>Tea, loose-leaf chai, green, ginger, mate, <2 cups/ day | Alcohol: mezcal, tequila, vodka, wine (biodynamic, low-sulfite): 10 drinks/week<br>Cranberry juice, pure, unsweetened<br>Fruit juice, from Mild fruit category<br>Green juice‡<br>Kombucha, low-sugar: <½ cup/day<br>Orange juice, fresh: ½ cup<br>Seltzer/carbonated beverages: ≤2 cups/day |
| **SWEETENERS** | | |
| Honey,* alfalfa, cotton, clover, raspberry: <1 tablespoon<br>Monk fruit, pure (no erythritol)<br>Stevia, pure (no inulin): in small amounts, occasionally | Allulose§<br>Brown rice syrup, rice malt syrup<br>Honey,* blackberry, buckwheat, orange blossom: 1 tablespoon<br>Sorghum syrup | Coconut sugar<br>Date sugar<br>Honey,* acacia, sage, tupelo<br>Maple syrup<br>Molasses<br>Polyols/sugar alcohols: isomaltol, erythritol, lactitol, maltitol, mannitol, sorbitol, xylitol: in small amounts, occasionally |

‡ The best green juices are freshly pressed with organic ingredients and no added sugar.
§ Limit allulose intake to <24 grams per serving or <54 grams per day to avoid GI symptoms.
* May need to avoid if fructose-intolerant.

## Dairy and Your Gut—What's Best?

Dairy has become controversial over the last two decades because, although it is touted as a healthy food and integral part of the food pyramid, at least 55 percent of the world's population has trouble digesting dairy products, and the prevalence of cow's milk allergy has been growing worldwide.[1] For many, eating dairy causes bloating, indigestion, nausea, gas, and other gut-centric symptoms.

Unlike twenty years ago, when having a lactose or dairy intolerance or allergy meant abstaining from anything even remotely milk-like, there are tons of options for you today. Dairy-free milks and other dairy product alternatives have skyrocketed in popularity, because cow's milk can be *allergenic* (allergy-provoking) and is (among the various dairy options) the most likely to cause food sensitivities and lactose intolerance. These days people are consuming products made of goat milk, sheep milk, camel milk, oat milk, almond milk, coconut milk, hemp milk . . . and the list keeps growing. Generally speaking, if you have issues drinking cow's milk, chances are there's a milk alternative out there that will give you less trouble.

That said, if you are hesitant to give up cow's milk products entirely or seem to tolerate them without major issues, I recommend you opt for a fermented milk product as specified in the food list above or raw cow's milk cheese.

As for which dairy alternatives will sit best with you, first check the food list in this chapter, then start testing small quantities based on your GutSMART Score and noting how you react. While some studies have been done to see which milks are most likely to elicit an immune response, there's no all-encompassing conclusion. In 2018, a study was done with several kinds of milk to determine which ones were most *immunoreactive or allergenic*, meaning which ones evoked the greatest immune system response.[2] The milks studied were cow, goat, sheep, camel, human, soy, almond, and coconut. Here's what researchers found:

- If an individual was immunoreactive to cow's milk, the probability of them being immunoreactive to goat and sheep milk was high. In other words, if they didn't tolerate cow's milk well due to a food sensitivity (not necessarily lactose intolerance), they were likely to not tolerate sheep or goat milk either.

- For those allergic to cow's milk, the *least allergenic* alternatives (the ones least likely to cause an immune reaction), in descending order, were human, camel, sheep, and goat milk.

- Of the plant-based milks tested, almond milk was the *most allergenic*, while coconut was the least.

While these findings are certainly useful in terms of providing you with direction, every person is different. Some people don't tolerate cow's milk well, but find other animal-derived milks to be no issue. They may also better tolerate milk from "A2" cows as opposed to "A1" cows (the most common type) because of a difference in the molecular structure of the casein protein that makes it easier to digest. Similarly, some people react poorly to specific plant-based milks.

In general, however, there are a few milk alternatives that may be easier for you to digest.[3]

If you don't have serious issues with cow's milk, try:

- Sheep milk

- Goat milk

- Organic kefir (a fermented yogurt-like beverage made from cow's milk)

If cow's milk is causing you to have symptoms (like gas, bloating, and diarrhea, or even constipation), try:

· Hemp milk

· Coconut milk

· Cashew milk

· Almond milk

· Oat milk

· Rice milk

*Note*: Many of the plant-based milks you find at the store contain ingredients that aren't gut-friendly, like gums, thickeners, and preservatives. These are added to improve and stabilize the texture of the milk, making it last longer. If you're going to buy your milk alternative at the store, you want to look for one that is unsweetened, carrageenan-free, and has very few ingredients (the fewer the better—for example, look for nuts, water, and salt only).[‡] What I encourage you to do, though, is make your own plant-based milks at home (see the recipes for homemade almond milk, page 172, and macadamia milk, page 173). It's *so* easy and in most cases more cost-effective than buying packaged milk—and in my opinion, tastes better, too!

In short, the best milk for your gut is the one that you can consume with no consequences, meaning no symptoms—either gut-centric, like digestive issues, gas, bloating, diarrhea, or constipation, or gut-related, like migraines, headaches, nasal or sinus congestion, brain fog, or fatigue. Follow the guidelines in the food list, but also *listen to your gut*.

---

[‡] One brand I particularly like is Elmhurst (see Elmhurst1925.com) because their plant-based milks are made with minimal ingredients and without gums, fillers, or emulsifiers.

# FOODS THAT SOOTHE & HEAL THE GUT

For those of you who tested Moderate or Severe in the GutSMART Quiz, there are a few foods I want to highlight that are standouts for healing and soothing the gut. Most, if not all, people tolerate these foods and spices well—so I encourage you to add them to your meals when you can in moderation!

### *Ginger*

Ginger has long been used as a medicine for gastrointestinal disorders and ailments, including constipation, diarrhea, belching, bloating, gastritis, abdominal discomfort, indigestion, and nausea.[4] There are tons of ways to use ginger, either fresh or in powdered form, but I recommend adding freshly grated ginger to your meals when it makes sense flavor-wise, or steeping a piece of fresh ginger in boiling water for ten minutes to make ginger tea to sip on.

### *Turmeric*

Turmeric's anti-inflammatory properties are well studied, and it's been shown to soothe digestive disorders, including irritable bowel syndrome (IBS) and inflammatory bowel disorder (IBD).[5] Similar to ginger, turmeric can be added in fresh or powdered form to savory recipes or made into a tea for an earthy, digestive relief. When adding turmeric powder to meals, make sure to sprinkle in some ground black pepper as well; black pepper increases absorption of the anti-inflammatory curcuminoids in turmeric.

### *Aloe*

When we think about aloe, it's usually in the context of healing burns, but aloe has digestive benefits, too, especially for those suffering from constipation, IBS, IBD, or stomach ulcers.[6] Aloe vera juice can be used as a natural laxative, and it can also help balance the microbiome by functioning like a *prebiotic* (explained below). Many of my clients add a tablespoon of store-bought aloe vera juice to their smoothies or just drink a shot of it. Be forewarned, though: Aloe vera juice is powerful. Start with one tablespoon, increase in small amounts, and use it only when your gut needs a reset, like when you're backed up.

### *Fennel*

Fennel is a digestion-friendly food we don't talk about often enough! Chewing fennel seeds is common in the Indian subcontinent, where it is used to aid digestion and prevent gas post-meals, but almost every part of the fennel plant is edible and good for the gut.[7] The easiest way to eat fennel bulb is to chop it, toss it in olive oil, and roast at 400°F for about twenty minutes, but you can also use it in sauces, soups, stews—you name it. And the fronds can easily be tossed into salads.

## Making Beans More Gut Friendly

Beans—a category that includes traditional black and kidney beans as well as legumes like chickpeas, lentils, and soybeans—are generally considered great for the gut. They're filled with fiber, after all! But contrary to popular belief, beans don't play nice with every gut. This is because beans—especially raw beans—contain high levels of gut disruptors called *lectins*.

Put simply, **lectins** are sugar-binding proteins that find their way to the simple sugars found on the cell surfaces of many tissues and attach to them. Researchers believe that by binding to these tissues, including the tissues of internal organs and glands like the thyroid, lectins can potentially trigger an immune response, leading to inflammation and even autoimmune disease.[8] In some instances, lectin-containing foods (like red kidney beans) have sent people to the ER with nausea and vomiting. If you are lectin-intolerant, you may experience digestive issues even when you eat cooked beans, including canned varieties.

Does this mean—assuming you aren't lectin-intolerant—you have to cut out beans altogether? Not necessarily. Most beans are not prepared in a gut-friendly fashion. (For this reason, beware of canned beans!) Preparing them properly can help! And the healthier your gut is, the easier it is to digest beans.

Start with dried lentils and beans, then soak them properly and cook them. Both soaking and cooking lower the lectin content of beans, making them more gut-friendly. **You should soak them in a bowl or pot of water overnight (or for at least eight hours).** However, *I recommend not soaking beans for longer than twelve hours, to keep the beans from taking on too much water.* And make sure not to leave your beans soaking for more than twenty-four hours (unless you are sprouting your beans); that's when the beans will start to ferment, altering their flavor profile and potentially making them *gut-unfriendly*, especially if you're in the Severe or Moderate category.

Any cooking method you use will reduce the lectin content, as long as you cook the beans all the way through, but my favorite is pressure cooking, because it's super fast. (If you have an Instant Pot, you only need to cook your beans on high heat for about ten minutes before they are safer to eat.) If you don't have a pressure cooker, you can reduce the lectin content by boiling your beans instead; you'll just need more time (anywhere from thirty minutes to two hours).

If you're cooking your beans on the stove, I recommend adding baking soda or **kombu** (a sea vegetable) to help soften the beans and make them even more digestible. Kombu contains the enzyme *alpha-galactosidase*, which acts as a natural bean tenderizer and breaks down the raffinose sugars (the gas-producing culprits) in beans. When you bring your beans and water to a boil, add ¼ teaspoon of baking soda or a piece of kombu the size of a postcard (or several thin strips) to your pot. Stir to combine and continue to cook as instructed. The baking soda will dissolve into the water and the kombu will start to break down after an hour. If you see any extra pieces of kombu, you can either eat them or toss them out. Once you do that, just drain your beans or follow the recipe directions and enjoy!

# THE POWER OF FERMENTED FOODS

I want to take a moment here to talk about one of the most exciting new revelations in gut health: the power of fermented foods to not only heal the gut, but also improve your overall health.

When I say "fermented foods," I mean foods that live bacteria or yeast have been allowed to grow on or in, producing chemical changes in the food that make them more digestible, produce vitamins, and increase their shelf life. That may sound icky, but it's a good thing, I promise! Fermented foods increase microbiome diversity and drastically reduce inflammatory markers.[9]

Here's a quick list of my go-to favorite ferments (choose based on your food list category):

- Kimchi
- Sauerkraut (unpasteurized); kraut juice
- Pickles (ones that are fermented, not just pickled)
- Brine-cured olives
- Yogurt (ideally Greek, skyr, or labneh, but I also love nondairy coconut yogurt; look for yogurts without added sugar—plain is best!)
- Fermented cottage cheese (from organic, grass-fed cow's or goat milk, or a plant-based source)
- Kefir (ideally made from goat milk or plant-based nut milks, or else organic, grass-fed cow's milk)
- Miso (from organic, non-GMO soybeans)
- Kombucha (again, watch the sugar content; stick with low-sugar options)
- Sourdough bread (and I mean the real, seventy-two-hour fermented stuff)

## A Word of Caution on Fermented Foods

I'm not exaggerating when I say fermented foods are *powerful* tools for improving your gut microbiome and digestion. And for that reason, eating too much of them at once or throughout the day can backfire on you. An excessive intake of fermented foods can lead to gas, bloating, indigestion, and even diarrhea or mental fog . . . all symptoms you may be trying to correct and avoid. This is especially true if you have **histamine intolerance** due to an overproduction of histamine or an inability to break it down, which causes allergy-like symptoms that include nasal congestion, flushing, itchy skin, and headaches. Fermented foods can make those issues worse. Everyone is different and can tolerate different levels of ferments, but I cannot stress this enough: *take it slow.*

The three principles I give my patients when they start eating ferments: *start small, go slow, and be intuitive.* When it comes to fermented foods, you definitely don't want to jump in too quickly. When I interviewed Fermentationist Summer Bock while writing this book, she recommended that anyone new to ferments start by eating *just ¼ teaspoon daily.* This allows you to test it out and see how your body responds. Sometimes that's all people can tolerate!

Follow the food chart to know which ferments and at what quantities are okay to test based on your level of gut dysfunction. Remember, listen to what your body says is "okay" for it, even if that contradicts some of the recommendations in this book. Ultimately, how your body reacts is your best guide.

*If the GutSMART Quiz puts you in the Severe category, I'm sorry to say you won't be able to tolerate ferments just yet.* It's best to avoid them at this stage. Once you've moved into the Moderate category, you can start testing small amounts of fermented foods then. Don't worry; that's okay. Ferments are wonderful for your gut health, but bigger portions are not always better. In this case, less is more.

## WHAT ABOUT PROBIOTIC SUPPLEMENTS?

Food is the foundation of the GutSMART Protocol, but as a doctor and gut health guru, I have seen thousands of patients over more than two decades of service, and I know that supplements like probiotics also play a key and critical role in healing the gut and body. There's no question about it! I always recommend probiotics to anyone who struggles with chronic gut health issues, but just like fermented foods, taking probiotics requires some basic know-how, and if you're new to probiotics, it's generally best to start low and increase slowly.

If you're going to take a probiotic supplement, I recommend starting with a low-count, lactose-free (if possible) probiotic with at least 30 billion **CFUs** per capsule. CFUs, or *colony-forming units,* indicate the strength of the probiotic. They indicate the concentration of bacteria found in each serving size (generally one capsule). Probiotics supplements vary in terms of which strains of bacteria they contain, so make sure to look for one that has different strains of *Bifidobacterium* and *Lactobacillus*, which are among the strains of probiotic bacteria that have been most clinically researched and have proven health benefits.

If your GutSMART Quiz score is Severe, you may not be able to tolerate traditional probiotics because they may actually cause uncomfortable gas and bloating. However, you can try a spore-based probiotic, instead. Spore-based probiotics come from bacteria that live in the soil. They have several special properties that make them particularly helpful in healing a severely dysfunctional gut: (1) the ability to crowd out other bad bugs in the gut, (2) the production of antimicrobial peptides that kill off unwanted gut microbes, (3) the ability to improve and reverse leaky gut,[10] and (4) the ability to regulate the immune response. And because they are in spore form, which protects them from stomach acid, they can be administered at lower CFUs than traditional probiotics, while still being effective.

## PREBIOTICS: FERTILIZER FOR YOUR PROBIOTIC BACTERIA

Taking probiotics supplements is great, but they're only one piece of the puzzle. They won't do enough for your long-term gut health unless you're also eating enough *prebiotics*.[11]

**Prebiotics** are indigestible fibers found in many fruits, vegetables, and grains that researchers have found play a key role in restoring microbiome balance.[12] Though prebiotics are largely indigestible to humans (because we lack the enzymes to break these fibers down into usable carbohydrates), these complex carbs are completely "digestible" food for our gut flora and used as fuel to produce **essential short-chain fatty acids** (**SCFAs**), like *butyrate* (thus why SCFAs are called *postbiotics*, as you may recall from chapter 3). SCFAs allow colon cells to stay healthy, plus help prevent changes that could lead to cancer, increase insulin sensitivity, improve blood sugar levels, reduce inflammation, regulate the immune system, and even act as controllers of gene expression in the brain, affecting neuroplasticity. Even your brain needs SCFAs from your gut bacteria in order to run properly, learn, and store memories.

> Prebiotics are like "fish food" for your gut flora—they are happily gobbled up and used to produce the symbiotic nutrients we need for optimal health.

Prebiotics occur naturally in many foods—specifically fruits, vegetables, and legumes—but you can also buy them in supplement form. As supplements, you'll find them in health food stores, either individually or in combination with other supplements or probiotics, labeled as inulin, fructo-oligosaccharides (FOS), galacto-oligosaccharides (GOS), and resistant starch, to name a few.

---

### Prebiotic-Rich Foods*

| | |
|---|---|
| Avocados | Red kidney beans |
| Whole grains (like oats) | Chickpeas (aka garbanzo |
| Garlic | beans) |
| Onions, shallots, and | Chicory |
| scallions | Bananas |
| Leeks | Watermelon |
| Jerusalem artichokes (aka | Grapefruit |
| sunchokes) | Flaxseeds |
| Asparagus | Apples |
| Lentils | Jicama root |

\* Remember to check the GutSMART Protocol food list in this chapter to confirm which prebiotic foods are okay for you to include in your diet based on your GutSMART Score.

---

As with fermented foods and probiotics, if you're new to prebiotics, I urge you to start slow, with just ¼ teaspoon, increasing by only ¼ teaspoon every 3 to 4 days. (This is especially true when trying prebiotic supplements.) Consuming too many prebiotics too quickly can leave you feeling gassy and bloated, and by introducing them slowly, you can more easily gauge whether or when to back off on the dose to avoid abdominal bloating and pain. Fiber can also constipate if you increase your fiber intake *without* increasing your hydration. So start by adding a few of these foods to your diet each week, drink more water, and take note of how you feel. Your body will tell you what it likes (and doesn't like) if you listen!

Speaking of, let's talk more about the importance of listening to your body when eating, both during the 14-Day GutSMART Protocol and beyond.

## INTUITIVE EATING

While I've put together the lists in this chapter of what foods to eat and what foods not to eat, as well as more detailed food lists based on your GutSMART Score, there's no list of foods or set of recommendations that can apply to everyone at every single moment. Yes, the instructions I've laid out here will work for a large chunk of people—I'd go as far as to say the majority. But there will inevitably be *something* on the "eat" list that doesn't work for you personally.

Maybe you score a 275 on the GutSMART Quiz, which indicates a Moderate level of gut dysfunction. The Moderate list says you can eat a certain food—but when you do, you don't feel well. I want you to understand that these are recommendations, not hard-and-fast rules with no exceptions.

> Every individual is different. The way to make sure the GutSMART Protocol works the best it can for you is to try my recommendations *and* tune in to your own body.

In other words, if I say, "You can eat this," and your body is telling you, "No, you can't," don't overrule what your body is saying in favor of staying true to this book. That's not loyalty or discipline—it's nonsense. For example, if you add coconut oil to your food and you don't feel so great when you eat it, then stop eating coconut oil. Listening to your body is more important than anything else—including listening to me or anyone else. There is always going to be a little bit of individual variation in how people react to foods.

But intuitive eating is about more than paying attention to how you respond to certain foods. It's about really tuning in to your body and that inner knowing around foods that is already there inside each and every one of us and is simply waiting to be heard.

The way I see it, there are three different times in relation to eating that you want to tap into your intuition: *before* eating, *during* eating, and *after* eating.

### Before Intuition

This use of intuition happens before you start eating—hence the name—and it's about recognizing and staying true to your hunger cues rather than just following prescribed eating times. Historically, we have developed windows of time that we consider the "right" hours to eat. You know the ones: breakfast between 7 and 9 AM, lunch between 12 and 2 PM, and dinner between 6 and 8 PM. We've conditioned ourselves mentally to adhere to them, to the point where we're more likely to follow these social norms than listen to what our body is telling us or cave to pressure from family or friends to eat more than our bodies truly desire or need.

Practicing *Before Intuition* looks like this:

- Ignoring the internal and external pressure to eat when you're not hungry.
- Giving yourself permission to let your hunger dictate your behavior, rather than telling yourself "I *should* be eating right now" even though you're not hungry.

The goal of *Before Intuition* is to honor your body's hunger cues, and value those over everything else. If you're not hungry for lunch at noon, don't eat at noon. If you're hungry at 4 PM, eat at 4 PM. Envision your best friend or partner by your side right now. Imagine it's 10 PM, and they tell you they're hungry. Would you say to them, "You can't eat right now, it's not the right time"? Would you judge them for eating because it's not breakfast, lunch, or dinnertime? I really hope not! This is how I want you to think about treating yourself. Resist the urge to override your body's signals just because it's not a "socially accepted" time of day to eat. (However, do see the box that follows and "Intermittent [Intuitive] Fasting for Gut Health" below to understand why eating too late or out of synchrony with normal eating times more often than not is harmful for your gut and increases *insulin resistance*, as explained in chapter 3, leading to unwanted weight gain.)

## How Eating Times Affect the Gut & Your Health

Although you shouldn't ignore your body's hunger cues, having a regular eating window *does* help regulate your *gut's circadian rhythm*. Gut bacteria have their own *circadian rhythm*, and studies have shown that our feeding time exerts control over these bacterial clocks, influencing things like immune and metabolic function.[13] It's often better to skip a meal and fast if you're not hungry rather than eat at odd times every day (for example, eating lunch at 12 PM on one day, but not until 4 PM the next day and 1 PM the following), because eating at haphazard times throws off your gut's circadian rhythm. This encourages bad bugs to proliferate and scrambles your insulin signaling (as described on page 63). Also, try not to eat too close to when you go to bed. Doing so will make your digestion sluggish and uncomfortable and interrupt the quality of your sleep. *Aim to finish eating your last meal at least three to four hours before bedtime.*

### During Intuition

*During Intuition* is meant to happen while you're eating, and it's about recognizing when you're full. When we eat mindlessly or emotionally, and/or don't practice *Before Intuition*, it's difficult to tap into our *During Intuition*. In this state, we're disconnected from our body and tend to override its signals.

In each of these types of intuition, it's important to think in terms of internal signals versus external expectations. Slow yourself down, follow the breathwork exercises in chapter 11,‡ and ask yourself what's driving you to eat. Is it hunger? Is it the situation or context you're in (a party, a

---

‡ The exercises in the Breathwork chapter from Sachin Patel and Amanda Gilbert are *stellar* ways to practice honing your *During Intuition*.

restaurant)? Or the fact that everyone else is still eating?

Embodying your *During Intuition* looks like this:

- Being as present and conscious as possible when you eat—not watching TV, scrolling on your phone, or being otherwise distracted—and chewing your food intentionally.
- Stopping between bites, putting your utensils down, and assessing your hunger level and how you feel throughout the meal so you know when to stop.

- Not letting the behavior of others around you dictate what you do. If you don't want another bite or piece of something, don't have one. What everyone else does has nothing to do with you.

The goal of *During Intuition* is to hear and respect your body when it says, "You're full, you can stop." It also means listening to body cues that may come up while you're eating that a certain food is not agreeing with you (see the next section for some of those clues).

### Snacking Between Meals & Your Gut

Although there are times when you may find it's necessary to have a snack between meals to keep your energy up or your blood sugar steady, as I talk about further below, under "Intermittent (Intuitive) Fasting for Gut Health," giving your gut a break allows for repair and a metabolic reset. It's preferable to eat well-balanced meals, ideally composed of 25 percent protein, 30 percent healthy fats, and 45 percent complex carbs, that give you enough nutrients to allow you to not eat between meals.

However, if you are looking for a gut-friendly snack between meals, start by checking the foods listed in this chapter as permitted under your specific GutSMART Quiz score. Examples of healthy snacks include foods in one of the following categories:

- Low-carb, high-fat (such as sprouted nuts and seeds)

- High-protein (such as a piece of wild salmon or dairy, if allowed)

- High-fiber, low-sugar (such as berries or greens)

Healthy daytime snacks should satiate your hunger without making you feel too full, so that you can digest them quickly, get the energy you need to keep going, and still have the desire to eat a regular, well-balanced meal later in the day.

### After Intuition

Last but not least is *After Intuition*. Of the three types, this may be the one you're most familiar with—it may have been the reason you picked up this book in the first place! *After Intuition* is about paying attention to whether foods sit well with you after you eat them or not.

Like the other two types of intuition, *After Intuition* requires you to listen to and connect with your body. Practicing it means:

- Keeping an eye out for gut-centric symptoms after eating, like abdominal pain, bloating, diarrhea, constipation, burping, flatulence, and cramping.
- Thinking about any gut-related symptoms you've been experiencing, and taking note of when they tend to flare up. Do they seem to happen more frequently after you've eaten a certain food? Look for patterns.

The goal of *After Intuition* is to discover patterns in how you feel after eating certain foods (tired, energetic, depressed, anxious, wired, irritated) and even how you look after eating them (perhaps you're bloated or your acne or rosacea flare up).

Bottom line: I don't want you to blindly follow my lists—or my meal plans!—without reservation. *I want you to use your intuition!* When you utilize these three types of intuition, you'll be shocked by how quickly you're able to start making more intuitive food choices, avoid overeating, and discover what foods work for your body and which don't.

## Intermittent (Intuitive) Fasting for Gut Health

While this is not a book about fasting (for that, I recommend my friend Will Cole's book, *Intuitive Fasting*), I do want to briefly mention the role of fasting in relation to the GutSMART Protocol and healing the gut.

When you fast, different gut bacteria become metabolically active that allow your gut lining to repair itself, while modulating and quieting the immune response. That's why, to fortify your gut-healing journey, I recommend developing an eating schedule that allows you to **fast for at least twelve hours every night between dinner and breakfast**. This type of fasting is an important component of the GutSMART Protocol and, by allowing your digestive system the time it needs to rest and repair itself, will accelerate your path to total gut-body-brain wellness.

What does this look like in practice? If you finish eating dinner at 7:30 PM, don't eat again until breakfast at 7:30 AM the following morning. (This also ensures you stop eating my recommended three to four hours before bedtime.)

Of course, this means **no eating whatsoever after dinner**. And I can already hear you thinking, *You mean no late-night chips?!* That can be tough when you've developed a habit of giving in to the midnight munchies. Hey, no judgment! I've been there!

Late-night cravings tend to happen for two reasons: *(1) habit*—you've conditioned your body to expect a snack at that hour of the night, or *(2) anxiety/stress*—they're often a sign that your work-life balance is off kilter and you aren't getting enough self-care. The first reason can be easily reprogrammed within two to three weeks by using the hacks I share below. The second means you need to devote more time to self-care. Once your nervous system is rebalanced using the strategies and tools in Part IV of this book, late-night cravings will become a thing of the past. It's that simple.

Here are my *hacks for conquering the late-night snacking habit.* When late-night cravings strike, instead of eating, try:

· Drinking a calming herbal tea, like chamomile or kava.

· Eating berries or an apple, orange, or banana.

· Doing 10 to 15 minutes of deep breathing exercises (see chapters 10 and 11).

· Just waiting 15 to 20 minutes—cravings come like the surge of a wave, and that time frame is typically all it takes for a craving to pass.

# READY TO START YOUR PERSONALIZED 14-DAY GUTSMART PROTOCOL?

You've done the prep work, understand the foundations of gut health, figured out your GutSMART Score, and learned the ins and outs of what to eat to heal your gut, along with some helpful tips and tricks. Now it's time to get started!

I introduced the GutSMART Protocol last chapter, but here's a refresher:

You're going to follow the GutSMART Protocol for fourteen days (two weeks). For each GutSMART category—Mild, Moderate, and Severe—I've put together an accompanying meal plan with the help of chef and clinical nutritionist Lee Holmes, which you'll find in the next chapter. Each plan is fourteen days long and is complete with recipes Lee and I have developed to be both delicious and gut-friendly. You can choose to follow the meal plan for your category exactly, but you can still be successful with the GutSMART Protocol even if you don't. Use as much or as little of each meal plan as you desire, as long as you stick to the general guidelines and foods listed for your GutSMART Score category. Feel free to use the recipes as inspiration to create your own meal plan, following the general advice in this chapter, the recommendations in your category's food list, and the inner intuitive eating wisdom you are developing and practicing.

Then, at the end of the fourteen days, I want you to take the GutSMART Quiz again, for two reasons. *First*, it's going to show you how far you've come (which will encourage you to go further!), and *second*, it's going to guide you as to your next steps (repeating the 14-day GutSMART Protocol based on your updated score).

### The GutSMART Protocol

1. Take the GutSMART Quiz and calculate your GutSMART Score.

2. Follow the GutSMART Protocol for 14 days (two weeks).

3. Take the GutSMART Quiz again, see where you are, and re-evaluate.

4. Repeat the GutSMART 14-day Protocol based on your new GutSMART Score.

5. Repeat until you reach your lowest score possible and love how you feel.

Remember, you can follow this sequence as many times as you desire to get to your goal. The lower you can get your score on the GutSMART Quiz, the better!

Healing your gut is a process—it takes commitment—but I can guarantee it's worth committing to because it will change your life.

Like one satisfied fan, Jean Louise, wrote: *"After 30 days on [Dr. Pedre's protocol], I got my life back. I was once again the person I knew I could be; clear thinking, energetic, balanced, ache-free . . . and best of all, back in control of who I am."*

And hey, *if you do the protocol one or more times and have some gut-related issues that you still need to work on, here's how you can continue your healing*: Head to the **Appendix** at the end of the book, where I share *how to fully reboot your gut* with a doctor-designed supplement-based plan that will also boost your overall well-being, like thousands before you have done under my guidance.

Woo-hoo! It's time to get started!

# PART III

# THE GUTSMART KITCHEN

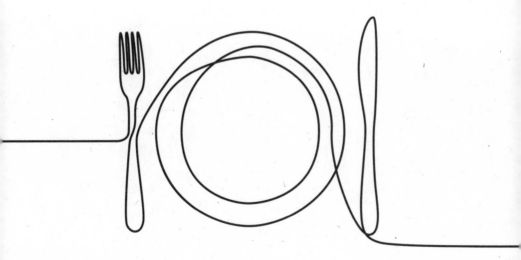

# Chapter 8

# MEAL PLANS

**The three meal plans detailed in this chapter are designed to com-**
plement your GutSMART Quiz score and where you are in your gut-healing journey. Like your GutSMART Score, they are divided into three categories: Mild, Moderate, or Severe.

Each meal plan covers fourteen days, and can be repeated as needed. (As you'll recall, you should retake the quiz upon completing each fourteen-day protocol to see where you stand.) As a reminder: By no means do these meal plans need to be followed exactly as written. I don't expect you to follow them to a T for every meal of every day. (For example, you are not expected to eat dessert every day!) In addition, you can adapt these plans to go with any style of eating, whether keto, paleo, Mediterranean, vegan, or vegetarian—as long as you follow the tips, comply with the food categories, and develop the intuitive eating skills described in chapter 7.

And hey, we're all human. I recognize you live in the real world, and in the real world, an endless number of things can come up that prevent you from sticking to any plan exactly as it's written. That's why I created the **What to _Enjoy_ Eating** (page 117) and **What to _Avoid_ Eating & Drinking** (page 119) lists as broad guidelines to follow, along with the more detailed GutSMART Food List—they'll help you make informed, empowered choices in the real world while still working towards gut bliss. I encourage you to grab a free digital copy of these resources and keep them with you at all times as a reference when eating out by going to **GutSMARTProtocol.com.**

Over the years, patients have often expressed to me their fear that eating gut-healthy will be "boring." Well, Chef Lee Holmes and I are here to show you that this is far from the truth! I'm so excited for you to experience the range of meals we've put together for you. And be sure to check out the next chapter, not only for all the recipes listed in these meal plans, but also for additional recipes and inspiration. These meal plans provide only a small peek at the vibrant, exciting food options that await you while you're working on healing your gut. And be sure not to miss the recipe pictures in the color insert; they're sure to entice you to be adventurous and make the delicious dishes we've carefully crafted for you!

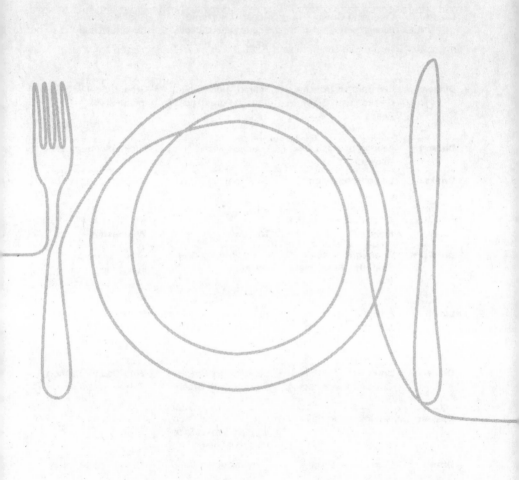

# MEAL PLAN: SEVERE

| Week One | | | |
|---|---|---|---|
| | **Monday** | **Tuesday** | **Wednesday** |
| **Breakfast** | Green Cleanse Smoothie | Overnight Protein Smoothie Bowl (make the night before) | Creamy Avocado Smoothie |
| **Lunch** | Cleansing Green Minestrone | Roasted Butternut Squash and Carrot Soup | Cool & Calming Coconut Soup |
| **Dinner** | Lemongrass Poached Chicken with Green Beans | Seared Tuna with Squash Puree and Herbs | Ground Beef with Peas Indian Style |
| **Dessert** | handful of nuts from Allowed list | 1 banana, sliced | ⅔ cup blueberries |
| **Drinks** | Lamb Bone Broth | Gut-Balancing Tonic | Chicken Bone Broth |
| **Week Two** | | | |
| | **Monday** | **Tuesday** | **Wednesday** |
| **Breakfast** | Overnight Protein Smoothie Bowl (make the night before) | Good Morning Green Smoothie | Green Cleanse Smoothie |
| **Lunch** | Baked Super Green & Berry Salad with Macadamia Dressing | Baked Papaya, Labneh, Brown Rice, and Pine Nut Salad | Stuffed Sweet Peppers with Lamb |
| **Dinner** | Snow Pea, Zucchini & Coconut Casserole | Lemongrass Poached Chicken with Green Beans | Wild-Caught Salmon Cakes |
| **Dessert** | ½ cup blueberries | leftover Baked Papaya, Labneh, Brown Rice & Pine Nut Salad | 1 kiwifruit |
| **Drinks** | Lamb Bone Broth | Gut-Balancing Tonic | Chicken Bone Broth |

| Week One | | | |
|---|---|---|---|
| **Thursday** | **Friday** | **Saturday** | **Sunday** |
| Good Morning Green Smoothie | Berry Beautiful Smoothie | Warm Savory Breakfast Bowl | Blue Breakfast Smoothie |
| Anti-Inflammatory Chicken & Veggie Soup | Stuffed Sweet Peppers with Lamb | Wild-Caught Salmon Cakes | Sweet Herb-Roasted Carrots + Crunchy Kaleslaw with Lime & Sesame Dressing |
| Roasted Root Vegetable Bowl with Aminos & Dulse Vinaigrette | Aromatic Chicken Curry | Grass-Fed Lamb with Broccoli Mash | Roasted Root Vegetable Bowl with Aminos & Dulse Vinaigrette |
| handful of nuts from Allowed list | 1/2 cup blueberries | Kiwi & Pineapple Rice Pudding | 1 kiwifruit |
| Tropical Mocktail | Gut-Balancing Tonic | Tropical Mocktail | Gut-Balancing Tonic |
| Week Two | | | |
| **Thursday** | **Friday** | **Saturday** | **Sunday** |
| Creamy Avocado Smoothie | Berry Beautiful Smoothie | Warm Savory Breakfast Bowl | Overnight Protein Smoothie Bowl (make the night before) |
| Baked Super Green & Berry Salad with Macadamia Dressing | Mixed Broth & Ginger Soup | Good Gut Falafel Grazing Board with Dips | Bunless Grass-Fed Beef Burger + Crispy Sweet Potato Fries |
| Ground Beef with Peas Indian Style | Seared Tuna with Squash Puree & Herbs | Aromatic Chicken Curry | Snow Pea, Zucchini & Coconut Casserole |
| handful of nuts from Allowed list | 1 banana, sliced | Kiwi & Pineapple Rice Pudding | 1 kiwifruit |
| Tropical Mocktail | Gut-Balancing Tonic | Tropical Mocktail | Gut-Balancing Tonic |

# MEAL PLAN: MODERATE

| Week One | | | |
|---|---|---|---|
| | **Monday** | **Tuesday** | **Wednesday** |
| **Breakfast** | Hazelnutty Banana Smoothie (make and freeze the night before) | Blue Breakfast Smoothie | Prickly Pear Oat Bowl |
| **Lunch** | Leek & Coconut Soup | Bunless Grass-Fed Beef Burger + Crispy Sweet Potato Fries | Mixed Broth & Ginger Soup |
| **Dinner** | Flaxseed-Crusted Wild-Caught Salmon | Fish & Lime Curry | Stuffed Sweet Peppers with Lamb |
| **Dessert** | berries with ¼ cup coconut yogurt | fresh fruit from Allowed list | Berry-Lime Pudding |
| **Drinks** | Digestive Green Shot | chai tea | 8 ounces coconut water |
| Week Two | | | |
| | **Monday** | **Tuesday** | **Wednesday** |
| **Breakfast** | Overnight Protein Smoothie Bowl (make the night before) | Good Morning Green Smoothie | Hazelnutty Banana Smoothie (make and freeze the night before) |
| **Lunch** | Broccoli & Peas with Hazelnuts, Lemon & Mint | Baked Papaya, Labneh, Brown Rice & Pine Nut Salad | Stuffed Sweet Peppers with Lamb |
| **Dinner** | Fish & Lime Curry | Gut-Balancing Veggie Stew | Beef Pho with Zucchini Noodles |
| **Dessert** | fresh fruit from Allowed list | 1 banana, sliced, with ¼ cup Greek yogurt | Berry-Lime Pudding |
| **Drinks** | Gut-Balancing Tonic | Digestive Green Shot | 8 ounces coconut water |

| Week One | | | |
|---|---|---|---|
| **Thursday** | **Friday** | **Saturday** | **Sunday** |
| Green Cleanse Smoothie | Berry Beautiful Smoothie | Creamy Avocado Smoothie | Blue Breakfast Smoothie |
| Baked Papaya, Labneh, Brown Rice & Pine Nut Salad | Wild-Caught Salmon Cakes | Boneless Grass-Fed Beef Burger | Spanish Jamon Serrano Frittata |
| leftover Fish & Lime Curry | Beef Pho with Zucchini Noodles | Roasted Quail with Root Veggies | Roasted Root Vegetable Bowl with Aminos & Dulse Vinaigrette |
| leftover Baked Papaya | Berries Served with Coconut Yogurt | Kiwi & Pineapple Rice Pudding | 1 banana, sliced, with ¼ cup Greek yogurt |
| Gut-Balancing Tonic | 2 ounces aloe vera juice | Digestive Green Shot | Tropical Mocktail |
| Week Two | | | |
| **Thursday** | **Friday** | **Saturday** | **Sunday** |
| Creamy Avocado Smoothie | Blue Breakfast Smoothie | Warm Savory Breakfast Bowl | Prickly Pear Oat Bowl |
| Baked Super Green & Berry Salad with Macadamia Dressing | Mixed Broth & Ginger Soup | Spanish Jamon Serrano Frittata | Bunless Grass-Fed Beef Burger + Crispy Sweet Potato Fries |
| Flaxseed-Crusted Wild-Caught Salmon | Lemongrass Poached Chicken with Green Beans | Grass-Fed Lamb with Broccoli Mash | Snow Pea, Zucchini & Coconut Casserole |
| pili nut yogurt | fresh fruit from Allowed list | Kiwi & Pineapple Rice Pudding | Fermented Berries with Coconut or Greek Yogurt |
| rooibos tea | Digestive Green Shot | Tropical Mocktail | chai tea |

# MEAL PLAN: MILD

| Week One | | | |
|---|---|---|---|
| | **Monday** | **Tuesday** | **Wednesday** |
| **Breakfast** | Happy Gut Granola | Chocolate & Berry Smoothie | Hazelnutty Banana Smoothie (make and freeze the night before) |
| **Lunch** | Grass-Fed Lamb Lettuce Leaf Tacos | Leek & Coconut Soup | Flaxseed-Crusted Wild-Caught Salmon |
| **Dinner** | Gut-Balancing Veggie Stew | Flaxseed-Crusted Wild-Caught Salmon | Lemongrass Poached Chicken with Green Beans |
| **Dessert** | Lemon & Berry Gelato | Nutty Apple Crumble | Berry-Lime Pudding |
| **Drinks** | Virgin Passion Fruit Mojito | Digestive Green Shot | Tropical Mocktail |
| Week Two | | | |
| | **Monday** | **Tuesday** | **Wednesday** |
| **Breakfast** | Good Morning Green Smoothie | Warm Savory Breakfast Bowl | Happy Gut Granola |
| **Lunch** | Spiced Roast Butternut Squash & Leftover Lamb Salad | Cleansing Green Minestrone | Bunless Grass-Fed Beef Burger + Crispy Sweet Potato Fries |
| **Dinner** | Beef Pho with Zucchini Noodles | Seared Tuna with Squash Puree & Herbs | Snow Pea, Zucchini & Coconut Casserole |
| **Dessert** | Kiwi & Pineapple Rice Pudding | Fermented Berries with Coconut or Greek Yogurt | Berry-Lime Pudding |
| **Drinks** | Gut-Balancing Tonic | Tropical Mocktail | Digestive Green Shot |

| Week One | | | |
|---|---|---|---|
| **Thursday** | **Friday** | **Saturday** | **Sunday** |
| Creamy Avocado Smoothie | Prickly Pear Oat Bowl | Happy Gut Granola | Slow-Scrambled Eggs, Mushrooms & Greens |
| Baked Super Green & Berry Salad with Macadamia Dressing | Anti-Inflammatory Chicken & Veggie Soup | Stuffed Sweet Peppers with Lamb | Goat Cheese, Sprouted Pumpkin Seed & Asparagus Salad |
| Beef Pho with Zucchini Noodles | Fish & Lime Curry | Roasted Root Vegetable Bowl with Aminos & Dulse Vinaigrette | Sunday Braised Lamb on Butternut Squash Mash |
| Fermented Berries with Coconut or Greek Yogurt | Kiwi & Pineapple Rice Pudding | Lemon & Berry Gelato | Nutty Apple Crumble |
| Gut-Balancing Tonic | Digestive Green Shot | Tropical Mocktail | herbal tea of choice |
| **Week Two** | | | |
| **Thursday** | **Friday** | **Saturday** | **Sunday** |
| Blue Breakfast Smoothie | Chocolate & Berry Smoothie | Overnight Protein Smoothie Bowl (make the night before) | Fermented Berries with Coconut or Greek Yogurt |
| Baked Super Green & Berry Salad with Macadamia Dressing | Goat Cheese, Sprouted Pumpkin Seed & Asparagus Salad | Good Gut Falafel Grazing Board with Dips | Baked Thyme Feta & Sardines with Buckwheat Crackers |
| Aromatic Chicken Curry | Roasted Quail with Root Veggies | Fish & Lime Curry | Sunday Braised Lamb on Butternut Squash Mash |
| Nutty Apple Crumble | Lemon & Berry Gelato | leftover Nutty Apple Crumble | Fermented Berries with Coconut or Greek Yogurt |
| Gut-Balancing Tonic | Digestive Green Shot | herbal tea of choice | Tropical Mocktail |

# Chapter 9

# RECItext

*"Eating for gut health doesn't have to be boring or bland. It can be a symphony of flavors with gut-healing ingredients that naturally repopulate the gut microbiome and balance the gut, so you can flourish and thrive."*

—Lee Holmes

**A symphony of flavors, indeed, is what chef and clinical nutritionist** Lee Holmes has put together for you in the recipes for *The GutSMART Protocol*. All you have to do is turn to the full-color recipe picture insert to get a sense of what eating right for your gut can look and feel like: a varied, colorful tour de force!

No, a gut-healing diet doesn't have to be boring, and yes, it can be sprinkled with a variety of flavors, colors, and smells to entice all of the senses—because whether you're just beginning your gut-healing journey or already halfway there, eating should be *fun*! And I can tell you that making these recipes has certainly been the highlight of many days for me. My sincere wish is that they become the highlight of your 14-Day GutSMART Protocol as well.

The recipes in this chapter are grouped into categories based on recipe type. Within each category, you'll find a mix of recipes for all three GutSMART Score categories: Severe, Moderate, and Mild. Remember, if you're in the Severe category, you can *only* eat the recipes marked Severe. If you scored Moderate, you can enjoy both the Severe and Moderate recipes. And if you scored Mild, you can enjoy all three categories of recipes—Severe, Moderate, and Mild. For this reason, we've included fewer recipes in the Moderate and Mild categories (17 Moderate and 17 Mild), and more in the Severe category (31). In total, we've included 65 recipes to choose from (with suggestions that allow you to adapt a few to other categories) as you embark on your culinary, gut-healing journey.

---

## GutSMART Tips

Throughout this chapter, you'll see some of my *GutSMART Tips*, little tips and tricks to help you make these delicious recipes with confidence. Here are a few to get you started.

- **A Soy Sauce Alternative?** Liquid coconut aminos can be used as a substitute for wheat-free tamari for anyone who needs or wants to avoid soy altogether.

- **Making Nuts and Seeds Easier on Your Gut:** Nuts and seeds, like almonds, cashews, pumpkin seeds, and sunflower seeds, have high levels of lectins and antinutrients (compounds that interfere with the body's absorption of nutrients), which irritate the gut lining and make them hard to digest. However, soaking them reduces these levels, making them easier to digest. For a more gut-friendly option, first soak nuts or seeds in filtered water for at least twelve hours. You can also drain and add fresh water every twelve hours until sprouted (typically 2 to 3 days), if desired, to activate their nutrients and make them even more gut-friendly.

- **Are Blended Raw Veggies Okay?** When blending raw vegetables, as in a smoothie, mocktail, or tonic, the blending process acts as a partial surrogate for digestion, making them easier to digest, even when raw. In recipes that call

---

for blending raw vegetables, just be sure to stick with those allowed in your category.

- **More Protein in Your Smoothie?** Protein is filling, and it also speeds up your metabolism like no other nutrient. I recommend adding a vegan protein powder (ideally micronized pea protein; see **GutSMARTProtocol.com** for options) to make your smoothie feel even more like a meal.

# CONTENTS

S Severe    M Moderate    M Mild

## Sensational Sides

## Fermented Delights

## Delectable Desserts

---

### Allergen Key

⊘ Contains nuts      ◌ Contains eggs      ⧘ Contains dairy

Recipes that offer an allergen-free substitution do not include an allergen icon.

---

Recipes with a 📷 also appear in the photo insert.

# SMOOTHIES & NONDAIRY MILKS

*Smoothies and nut milks are an easy way to facilitate the digestion and absorption of nutrients that otherwise might be hard to break down, especially for those with severe gut dysfunction. With smoothies, you can pack in a ton of nutrients that might be missed when eating other grab-and-go meals. I love starting my day with a smoothie.*

## Smoothie-Making Tip

I recommend always using a high-speed blender for making smoothies.‡ While high-speed blenders certainly make blending easier, following these steps even with a regular blender will simplify the process and ensure a well-blended smoothie:

1. Add the liquid ingredients.
2. Turn the blender on low, then add the powdered ingredients while the blender is blending. This keeps them from sticking to the sides.
3. Turn off the blender, then add the harder ingredients (like nuts, seeds).
4. Blend on high until smooth.
5. Add any greens, fruit, frozen ingredients, and ice.
6. Blend on high until smooth.
7. Pour into a tall glass, then add toppings and enjoy!

‡ My two favorite brands are Vitamix and Nutribullet.

## Green Cleanse Smoothie Ⓢ
Makes 1 to 2 servings

### INGREDIENTS

1 cup coconut water
½ cup almond milk (page 172 or store-bought) or hemp milk for nut-free alternative
½ teaspoon spirulina
1 small handful baby spinach leaves
4 kale leaves, stemmed
1 small cucumber, seeded
¼ large or ½ small avocado, pitted and peeled

### STEPS

Blend all the ingredients in a blender until smooth. Enjoy!

## Berry Beautiful Smoothie Ⓢ
Makes 1 to 2 servings

### INGREDIENTS

1 tablespoon lime juice
1½ cups macadamia milk (page 173 or store-bought) or hemp milk for nut-free alternative
1 teaspoon sprouted pumpkin seeds
1 teaspoon sprouted sunflower seeds
1 teaspoon grated lime zest
½ cup fresh or frozen mixed berries (including ≤10 strawberries, ≤10 raspberries, and ≤10 blueberries)
1 cup ice cubes or crushed ice

### STEPS

Blend all the ingredients in a blender until smooth. Enjoy!

## Creamy Avocado Smoothie ⓢ

Makes 1 serving

**INGREDIENTS**

¼ cup coconut water
¼ cup additive-free
   coconut milk, plus more
   if needed to achieve the
   desired texture
1 teaspoon honey
1 scoop pea or vegan
   protein
¼ medium avocado, pitted
   and peeled
1 small frozen banana, cut
   into chunks
1 cup ice cubes or crushed
   ice

**STEPS**

Blend all the ingredients in a blender until smooth.
Enjoy!

## Blue Breakfast Smoothie ⓢ

Makes 1 to 2 servings

**INGREDIENTS**

1½ cups macadamia milk
   (page 173 or store-
   bought) or hemp milk
   for nut-free alternative
½ teaspoon alcohol-free
   vanilla flavoring
1 teaspoon bee pollen,
   plus more for garnish
½ teaspoon blue spirulina
1 cup baby spinach leaves
   or ½ cup frozen spinach
1 frozen banana, cut into
   chunks, plus extra slices
   for garnish
¼ cup frozen raspberries
   (≤10)
½ cup ice cubes or
   crushed ice

**STEPS**

Blend all the ingredients in a blender until smooth.
Enjoy!

**GARNISH (OPTIONAL)**

Decorate with extra banana slices and bee pollen.

##  Good Morning Green Smoothie Ⓢ

Makes 1 large serving

### INGREDIENTS

⅔ cup almond milk (below, or store-bought) or hemp milk for nut-free alternative
1 tablespoon lemon juice
5 kale leaves, stemmed
Handful fresh arugula
1 small cucumber, seeded
¼ medium avocado, pitted and peeled
1 kiwifruit, peeled and cut into chunks
1 frozen or fresh banana

### STEPS

Blend all the ingredients in a blender until smooth. Enjoy!

## Almond Milk Ⓢ Ⓜ ⌗

Makes about 4 cups

### INGREDIENTS

1 cup blanched almonds
3 cups filtered water, boiled then cooled slightly
¼ teaspoon alcohol-free vanilla flavoring or vanilla powder
Stevia powder, up to 1 teaspoon (optional)*

*Adapt It: As a modification for Moderate (or Mild), you can substitute allulose for the stevia to sweeten the almond milk.

### STEPS

1. Blend the almonds, water, and vanilla in a blender until smooth.

2. Strain through a fine-mesh sieve, reserving the almond pulp to use again (see tip).

3. Sweeten the almond milk with stevia to taste and enjoy right away, or pour into an airtight sterilized container and keep refrigerated for up to 5 days.

**GutSMART Tip:** You can make more almond milk by adding the leftover almond pulp to the blender with more water (this can be done up to three times) and then straining it. The almond pulp will keep in a sealed container in the fridge for up to 3 days.

## Macadamia Milk Ⓢ Ⓜ 🔗

Makes 4½ cups

### INGREDIENTS

1 cup raw macadamia nuts
4 cups filtered water, boiled then cooled slightly
¼ teaspoon alcohol-free vanilla flavoring or vanilla powder
1 teaspoon stevia, or to taste*

***Adapt It:** As a modification for Moderate (or Mild), you can substitute allulose for the stevia.*

### STEPS

1. Combine all the ingredients in a high-speed blender and blend for 30 seconds, or until smooth.

2. Enjoy right away, or pour the milk straight into a sterilized airtight container—it doesn't need to be strained. It will keep in the fridge for up to 4 days.

## 📷 Hazelnutty Banana Smoothie Ⓜ 🔗

Makes 1 serving

### INGREDIENTS

⅔ cup almond milk (page 172 or store-bought)
1 teaspoon rice malt syrup or allulose
½ teaspoon alcohol-free vanilla flavoring
4 teaspoons almond butter
¼ cup hazelnuts, plus 1 hazelnut, chopped, for garnish
2 Brazil nuts
1 frozen banana, cut into chunks

### STEPS

1. Blend all the ingredients in a blender until smooth.

2. Pour into a glass and garnish with the chopped hazelnut. Enjoy!

## Chocolate & Berry Smoothie ⓜ

Makes 1 serving

### INGREDIENTS

1 cup almond milk (page
    172 or store-bought) or
    hemp milk for nut-free
    alternative
1 tablespoon chia seeds
1 tablespoon raw cacao
    powder
1 teaspoon raw cacao nibs,
    plus more for garnish
1 ripe banana
5 strawberries
⅔ cup blueberries
6 ice cubes

### STEPS

Blend all the ingredients in a blender until smooth.
Enjoy!

### GARNISH (OPTIONAL)

Top with cacao nibs for extra crunch.

# GRANOLA & BREAKFAST BOWLS

*Finding a gut-friendly breakfast can be challenging, but with these break-fast bowls and granola, along with the smoothies above, you are sure to enjoy a variety of options. A warm, savory breakfast bowl takes me back to my time visiting Thailand, where it is a common breakfast item. It's a great way to start the day. And the gut-friendly Happy Gut Granola (see color insert) also makes an excellent portable, go-to snack.*

## Overnight Protein Smoothie Bowl Ⓢ Ⓜ ⌗

Makes 1 large bowl

### INGREDIENTS

½ cup frozen or fresh mixed berries (blueberries, raspberries, and/or strawberries)

2 tablespoons sprouted sunflower seeds, plus more for garnish\*

1 scoop pea protein powder (see tip)

Grated zest of 1 small lime

1 tablespoon lime juice

½ cup almond milk (page 172 or store-bought)

½ cup additive-free coconut milk

2 teaspoons raw honey or 1 teaspoon monk fruit powder (optional)

1 teaspoon alcohol-free vanilla flavoring

1 tablespoon sprouted almonds, roughly chopped

1 teaspoon hemp seeds\*

*\*Adapt It: You can adapt this recipe for the Mild category by substituting equal portions of chia seeds for the sunflower seeds and hemp seeds.*

### STEPS

1. Combine all the ingredients (except the garnishes) in a glass jar or bowl and refrigerate overnight.

2. In the morning, pour the contents of the jar into a blender and blend until smooth.

3. Top with the sprouted almonds and a sprinkle of sprouted sunflower seeds and hemp seeds.

*GutSMART Tip: Pea protein isolate is one of the most gut-friendly protein powders you can use. Most people tolerate pea protein quite well, especially when it is micronized for easier digestion. You can find micronized pea protein powder in vanilla and chocolate flavors at GutSMARTprotocol.com.*

## 📷 Warm Savory Breakfast Bowl Ⓢ

Makes 2 servings

### INGREDIENTS

10 green beans, chopped
1 carrot, spiralized
3 kale leaves, stemmed
  and roughly chopped
1 cup cooked white rice
½ cucumber, seeded and
  diced, or ½ English
  cucumber, diced
¼ medium avocado,
  pitted, peeled, and
  sliced
1 (5-ounce) can fresh wild-
  caught sardines in extra
  virgin olive oil, drained
1 tablespoon extra virgin
  olive oil
1 tablespoon lemon juice
Sea salt and freshly
  ground black pepper,
  to taste
Fresh cilantro leaves, for
  garnish

### STEPS

1. Steam the green beans and carrot over boiling water for 5 minutes, or until just al dente, then add the kale and cook until it has wilted.

2. Transfer the vegetables to a bowl.

3. Add the rice and cucumber and stir to combine with the steamed vegetables.

4. Arrange the avocado and sardines on top.

5. Drizzle with the olive oil and lemon juice and season with salt and pepper. Garnish with cilantro and serve warm.

## Prickly Pear Oat Bowl Ⓜ

Makes 2 servings

### INGREDIENTS

2 prickly pears or 1 Asian pear, peeled and chopped

1½ teaspoons ground cinnamon, plus more for garnish

⅓ cup filtered water

1 cup organic gluten-free rolled oats (porridge)

2 cups additive-free coconut milk or hemp milk

¼ teaspoon vanilla powder

### STEPS

1. Combine the pears, cinnamon, and water in a small saucepan and bring to a boil.

2. Reduce the heat and simmer until the pears are soft, 5 to 8 minutes. Remove from the heat.

3. Meanwhile, in another saucepan, simmer the oats in the coconut milk for 12 to 15 minutes, or until the oats are tender, stirring regularly.

4. Stir the pears and vanilla powder into the oats and continue cooking for another 1 to 2 minutes.

5. Spoon into serving bowls. Sprinkle with extra cinnamon and serve.

## 📷 Happy Gut Granola ⓜ 🔗

Makes 8 to 10 servings

### INGREDIENTS

1½ cups quinoa or brown rice flakes

1 cup sulfite-free dried apricots, roughly chopped

¾ cup walnuts, chopped

3 tablespoons sprouted or dry-roasted sunflower seeds

2 tablespoons dried blueberries

2 tablespoons sprouted pumpkin seeds (pepitas)

2 tablespoons sliced almonds

1 tablespoon flaxseeds

½ teaspoon ground cinnamon

½ teaspoon freshly grated nutmeg

3 tablespoons extra virgin coconut oil

2 tablespoons rice malt syrup or maple syrup

½ teaspoon alcohol-free vanilla flavoring

¼ cup coconut flakes

1 tablespoon currants

### Garnish (per serving)

½ cup almond milk (page 172 or store-bought)

¼ cup blueberries

1 mint sprig

### STEPS

1. Preheat the oven to 350°F.

2. Combine the quinoa flakes, apricots, walnuts, sunflower seeds, dried blueberries, pumpkin seeds, almonds, flaxseeds, cinnamon, and nutmeg in a bowl and mix well to combine.

3. Heat the coconut oil in a small saucepan over medium heat until melted.

4. Add the rice malt syrup and vanilla and stir for 30 seconds. Remove from the heat.

5. Pour the liquid mixture over the dry ingredients and stir well, ensuring the dry ingredients are coated thoroughly.

6. Transfer the granola to a large rimmed baking sheet, in a single layer, and bake for 20 minutes, stirring frequently and breaking up any clumps that form.

7. Carefully remove the baking sheet from the oven, add the coconut flakes and currants, and bake for another 5 minutes.

8. Remove from the oven, let the mixture cool, and place in an airtight jar. Store in a cool, dry place for up to 1 month.

9. Combine ½ cup granola with the almond milk and top with fresh blueberries and a mint sprig. Enjoy!

**GutSMART Tip:** The Happy Gut Granola can be eaten as a stand-alone, as an on-the-go snack, or in a bowl with homemade almond or macadamia milk.

# MOCKTAILS & GUT TONICS

*Whenever you're on any sort of eating plan, one thing that is often missed is a nice cocktail. That's why I wanted to capture the adventure and surprise that comes with a well-crafted cocktail in these mocktails and gut tonics that I'm sure you will find delightful. The Tropical Mocktail (see color insert) is one of my favorites!*

## Tropical Mocktail Ⓢ

Makes 1 serving

### INGREDIENTS

1 passion fruit
½ cup coconut water
½ cup aloe vera juice
1 tablespoon lime juice
Handful ice cubes

### STEPS

1.  Cut the passion fruit in half and scoop the pulp and seeds into a glass.

2.  Add the coconut water, aloe vera juice, lime juice, and ice cubes, and stir gently.

> **GutSMART Tip:** *If passion fruit is not in season, you can substitute pineapple. Cut the pineapple into chunks and pop it in a blender to create a pineapple puree the consistency of passion fruit. Use ½ cup pineapple puree.*

## ⬚ Gut-Balancing Tonic Ⓢ

Makes 2 to 3 servings

**INGREDIENTS**

1 medium celery stalk, roughly chopped
1 large carrot, roughly chopped
1 medium cucumber, seeded and roughly chopped, or 1 medium English cucumber, roughly chopped
½ small fennel bulb, roughly chopped
2 cups coconut water
1 lime, peeled and roughly chopped
1 small handful fresh mint leaves
¼ cup aloe vera juice
1 probiotic capsule (optional)
1 teaspoon honey, monk fruit, or stevia to taste
Ice cubes, for serving

**STEPS**

1.  Combine the celery, carrot, cucumber, fennel, and coconut water in a high-speed blender and blend.

2.  Add the lime and mint leaves and blend until smooth.

3.  Stir in the aloe vera juice and the contents of the probiotic capsule, if using.

4.  Sweeten to taste and serve over ice.

## ⬚ Digestive Green Shot Ⓜ

Makes 2 servings

**INGREDIENTS**

1¼ cups filtered water
1 tablespoon lemon juice
15 baby spinach leaves
½ cup arugula
2 kiwifruits, peeled
2 English cucumbers, peeled and roughly chopped
2-inch knob ginger, peeled
1 handful flat-leaf parsley leaves and stems

**STEPS**

1.  Combine all the ingredients, in the order listed, in a high-speed blender. Blend until smooth.

2.  For a finer drink with no pulp, pour the mixture through a fine-mesh sieve, push it through with the back of a spoon, and strain into two glasses. Enjoy!

# Virgin Passion Fruit Mojito Ⓜ

Makes 4 servings

## INGREDIENTS

2 limes
1 passion fruit
1 handful mint leaves, plus
    more to garnish
1 teaspoon maple syrup
4 cups mineral water,
    divided (1 cup + 3 cups)
Crushed ice, for serving

## STEPS

1.  Grate the zest from 1 lime into a pitcher. Cut the zested lime into thin wedges and add to the pitcher.

2.  Cut the passion fruit in half and scoop the pulp and seeds into the pitcher. Add the mint and maple syrup.

3.  With a long-handled spoon or muddler, mash or stir the mixture gently, then pour about 1 cup of the mineral water into the pitcher. Pour slowly as it can become fizzy.

4.  Set aside to infuse for about 10 minutes.

5.  Meanwhile, cut the other lime into wedges and set aside for serving.

6.  Pour the mojitos into four tall glasses, then top up each glass with the remaining mineral water, again pouring slowly to avoid fizzing over.

7.  Top with crushed ice and garnish the glasses with extra mint and the reserved lime wedges. Enjoy!

### GutSMART Tips:

- If passion fruit is not in season, you can substitute mango (fresh or frozen).
- If mineral water is not available, you can substitute sparkling water, but be careful when pouring.

# BONE BROTHS & STOCKS

*Nothing conjures up gut-healing more than a delicious, warming bone broth, and homemade bone broth is like a pot of love for your gut. It can be sipped on its own or used as the foundation for other dishes. You can even substitute broth for water when making a side of rice to give it extra flavor.*

## GutSMART Tips:

- Bone broth can be made in a slow cooker. Cook on low for up to 24 hours, topping up with filtered water if it reduces too much.

- There will be a lot of fat, but it's okay to leave it there as it helps the broth keep longer in the refrigerator. If desired, you can skim off some of the fat to make it less dense.

- Leftover broth will keep in an airtight container in the refrigerator for up to 4 days or in the freezer for up to 1 month. You can even freeze it in ice cube trays to use to flavor recipes.

## Vegetable Broth Ⓢ

Makes 4 to 5 cups

### INGREDIENTS

3 carrots, roughly chopped

½ butternut squash, seeded and roughly chopped

1 celery root, peeled and roughly chopped

1 zucchini, roughly chopped

1 fennel bulb, roughly chopped

1 bunch scallions, green parts only, chopped

1 tablespoon extra virgin olive oil

1 small bunch flat-leaf parsley

4–5 thyme sprigs

1 bay leaf

1 tablespoon lemon juice

8 cups filtered water, or more as needed

Celtic sea salt and freshly cracked black pepper, to taste

### STEPS

1. Preheat the oven to 400°F.

2. Combine the carrots, butternut squash, celery root, zucchini, fennel, and scallions in a large roasting pan and splash with the olive oil, tossing to coat.

3. Roast for 45 minutes, stirring often. (You may have to remove the vegetables that cook faster as they are ready).

4. Transfer the roasted vegetables to a large stockpot. Add the parsley, thyme, bay leaf, and lemon juice. Season to taste with salt and pepper.

5. Add filtered water to cover and bring to a boil over medium heat.

6. Reduce the heat to low and simmer for 1 hour.

7. Carefully strain the broth through a cheesecloth-lined sieve into another pot or large bowl.

8. Serve right away, or let cool and store in an airtight container in the fridge for up to 4 days or in the freezer for up to 1 month.

## Lamb Bone Broth ⓢ

Makes 3 to 4 servings

### INGREDIENTS

¼ cup extra virgin coconut oil

4 ounces lamb marrow bones

8 cups filtered water, plus more as needed

2 carrots, peeled and roughly chopped

1 medium celery stalk, roughly chopped

1 bunch scallions, green parts only, chopped

1 bay leaf

2 tablespoons lemon juice

Celtic sea salt and freshly cracked black pepper, to taste

### STEPS

1. Preheat the oven to 400°F.

2. Melt the coconut oil in a 2½-quart casserole dish over medium heat.

3. Add the bones and stir to coat. Cover the casserole dish and transfer to the oven.

4. Roast for 30 minutes, or until the bones are browned.

5. Transfer the bones to a large stockpot, cover the bones with the filtered water, and add the remaining ingredients.

6. Bring to a boil on the stovetop, then reduce the heat to the lowest setting and simmer, uncovered, for 4 to 6 hours. Add a little more filtered water from time to time if necessary.

7. Remove from the heat and allow to cool, then strain through a fine-mesh sieve into a large bowl. Refrigerate until the fat congeals on top.

8. Skim off the fat if desired (although it does add flavor and helps preserve the broth) and store the stock in an airtight container in the fridge for up to 4 days or in the freezer for up to 1 month.

# Chicken Bone Broth Ⓢ

Makes 3 to 4 servings

## INGREDIENTS

1 whole organic chicken
2 chicken feet (for extra gelatin, optional)
8 cups filtered water, plus more as needed
¼ cup lemon juice
1 bunch scallions, green parts only, chopped
1 medium celery stalk, chopped
1 bay leaf
Celtic sea salt and freshly cracked black pepper, to taste
1 bunch flat-leaf parsley

## STEPS

1. In a large stockpot, combine the chicken, chicken feet (if using), water, lemon juice, scallions, celery, bay leaf, and salt and pepper.

2. Bring to a boil over medium heat, skimming off any foam that rises to the top.

3. Reduce the heat to the lowest setting, cover, and simmer for 2 hours.

4. Remove from the heat, and transfer the chicken to a cutting board. When cool enough to handle, take the meat off the bones, reserving the bones and setting aside the meat for another use.

5. Return the bones to the pot and simmer over very low heat, uncovered, for an additional 4 to 6 hours, checking from time to time and adding a little more filtered water if necessary.

6. About 10 minutes before removing from heat, add the parsley.

7. Remove the bones with a slotted spoon and allow the stock to cool. Strain the stock through a fine-mesh sieve into a large bowl and refrigerate until the fat congeals on top.

8. Skim off the fat if desired (although it does add flavor and helps preserve the broth) and store the stock in an airtight container in the fridge for up to 4 days or in the freezer for up to 1 month.

**GutSMART Tip:** The cooked chicken can be used in other recipes as needed or broken up into pieces and frozen for use at a later time.

## Gut-Friendly Mixed Broth (Beef, Lamb & Bison) Ⓜ

Makes 3 to 4 servings

### INGREDIENTS

¼ cup extra virgin
coconut oil

14 ounces lamb marrow
bones

14 ounces beef marrow
bones

7 ounces bison soup
bones

8 cups filtered water, or
more as needed

2 carrots, peeled and
roughly chopped

3 scallions, green parts
only, roughly chopped

1 bay leaf

2 tablespoons apple cider
vinegar

Celtic sea salt and freshly
cracked black pepper,
to taste

### STEPS

1. Preheat the oven to 400°F.

2. Melt the coconut oil in a 2½-quart casserole
   dish over medium heat.

3. Add the lamb, beef, and bison bones and stir to
   coat. Cover the casserole dish and transfer to
   the oven.

4. Roast for 30 minutes, or until the bones are
   browned.

5. Transfer the bones to a large stockpot, cover
   the bones with the filtered water, and add the
   remaining ingredients.

6. Bring to a boil on the stovetop, then reduce
   the heat to the lowest setting and simmer,
   uncovered, for 4 to 6 hours. Add a little more
   filtered water from time to time, if necessary.

7. Remove from the heat and allow to cool, then
   strain through a fine-mesh sieve into a large
   bowl. Refrigerate until the fat congeals on top.

8. Skim off the fat if desired (although it does add
   flavor and helps preserve the broth) and store
   the stock in an airtight container in the fridge
   for up to 4 days or in the freezer for up to 1
   month.

# NOURISHING SOUPS

*Soups, like bone broths, are like a warm hug for your gut. When the aromas of a soup fill the air in your kitchen, they get your salivary glands primed and your digestive juices going in anticipation. These soup recipes are all so good, it's hard to decide which is my true favorite, but the Roasted Butternut Squash & Carrot Soup and the Beef Pho with Zucchini Noodles are both exceptionally delicious and gut-soothing.*

> **GutSMART Tip:** *For all of these nourishing soups, you can store leftovers in the fridge for up to 4 days or in the freezer for up to 1 month.*

##  Roasted Butternut Squash & Carrot Soup Ⓢ 🔗

Makes 3 servings

### INGREDIENTS

¼ cup peeled butternut squash chunks
3 carrots, peeled and roughly chopped
1 teaspoon lemongrass powder or paste
1 teaspoon fennel seeds
1 star anise pod, broken up
1 tablespoon pine nuts, plus more for garnish
1 tablespoon extra virgin olive oil
4¼ cups vegetable broth (page 183 or store-bought)
Pinch grated lemon zest
2 tablespoons lemon juice
2 tablespoons wheat-free tamari or liquid coconut aminos for soy-free
Nutritional yeast, for garnish

### STEPS

1. Preheat the oven to 425°F.

2. Spread out the butternut squash and carrots on a rimmed baking sheet. Sprinkle the lemongrass, fennel seeds, star anise, and pine nuts over the top, then drizzle with the olive oil.

3. Bake for 30 minutes, or until golden.

4. Transfer the squash and carrots to a medium saucepan. Add the broth, lemon zest and juice, and tamari or liquid coconut aminos and bring to a gentle boil over medium heat.

5. Remove from the heat and let cool slightly, then blend in a blender until smooth.

6. Top with a sprinkle of nutritional yeast and extra pine nuts. Reheat if necessary and serve.

## Cleansing Green Minestrone ⑤

Makes 2 to 3 servings

### INGREDIENTS

1 tablespoon extra virgin
  olive oil
1 medium celery stalk,
  diced
1 carrot, peeled and diced
2 zucchinis, diced
1 large green bell pepper,
  diced
⅓ cup chopped kale
4 cups vegetable
  broth (page 183 or
  store-bought)
½ cup sprouted adzuki
  beans (soaked in warm
  water for 1 hour prior to
  cooking, then drained)
½ cup sprouted mung
  beans (soaked in warm
  water for 1 hour prior to
  cooking, then drained)
½ cup chopped fresh
  herbs, such as flat-
  leaf parsley, basil, or
  cilantro
½ cup sliced scallions,
  green parts only
¼ cup fresh or thawed
  frozen peas
Sea salt and freshly
  ground pepper, to taste

### STEPS

1. Heat the olive oil in a medium saucepan over low heat.

2. Add the celery and cook, stirring frequently, for 2 to 3 minutes, until softened.

3. Add the carrot, zucchinis, bell pepper, and kale, stirring to combine, and cook until softened, another 2 to 3 minutes.

4. Add the broth, sprouted adzuki, and mung beans and stir to combine.

5. Bring to a gentle boil, then simmer over low heat for 20 minutes.

6. Stir in the herbs, scallions, and peas and simmer for another 3 minutes.

7. Season to taste with salt and pepper. Serve.

**GutSMART Tip:** *Adzuki beans are the easiest to digest, but if they aren't available, either use just ½ cup sprouted mung beans or eliminate the beans altogether.*

## Cool & Calming Coconut Soup Ⓢ

Makes 2 servings

### INGREDIENTS

1 tablespoon extra
   virgin coconut oil or 2
   teaspoons grass-fed
   ghee
1 tablespoon chopped
   chives
½ cup chopped scallions,
   green parts only
¾ cup chopped zucchini
1 cup roughly chopped
   baby spinach
1 green bell pepper,
   seeded and diced
1 small handful watercress
   (about 12 leaves)
1 (9-ounce) can additive-
   free coconut milk
1 tablespoon lemon juice
2 cups finely chopped
   fresh herbs (such as
   basil, flat-leaf parsley,
   sage, dill, and tarragon)
1½ cups vegetable
   broth (page 183 or
   store-bought)
Celtic sea salt and freshly
   cracked black pepper,
   to taste
Chopped fresh cilantro,
   for garnish (optional)

### STEPS

1. Melt the oil in a medium saucepan over medium heat.

2. Add the chives and scallions and cook, stirring frequently, for 2 minutes, or until softened.

3. Add the zucchini, spinach, bell pepper, watercress, coconut milk, lemon juice, herbs, and broth and bring to a boil.

4. Reduce the heat to low, cover, and simmer for 20 minutes.

5. Remove from the heat and allow to cool slightly, then puree in a blender until smooth.

6. Season with salt and pepper and reheat if necessary.

7. Garnish with cilantro and serve.

## Anti-Inflammatory Chicken & Veggie Soup Ⓢ
Makes 3 to 4 servings

**INGREDIENTS**

1 tablespoon coconut oil
½ cup sliced scallions, green parts only
1 bunch kale, stemmed and roughly chopped
½ small broccoli head, roughly chopped
3½ ounces (three handfuls) baby spinach leaves
1 pound organic boneless, skinless chicken breasts, cut into bite-size pieces
Celtic sea salt and freshly cracked black pepper, to taste
½ cup chopped zucchini
2 carrots, peeled and diced
4 cups vegetable broth (page 183 or store-bought)
1 tablespoon nutritional yeast flakes
2 tablespoons wheat-free tamari or liquid coconut aminos for soy-free
1 tablespoon lemon juice

**STEPS**

1. Melt the oil in a large saucepan over medium heat.

2. Add the scallions and cook for 3 to 4 minutes.

3. Add the kale, broccoli, and spinach and cook for 3 to 4 minutes.

4. Season the chicken lightly with salt and pepper, then add to the pan, along with the zucchini and carrots. Cook, stirring frequently, for 5 minutes, or until the chicken is browned on all sides.

5. Pour in the broth and bring to a boil. Reduce the heat to low and cook for 10 minutes.

6. Add the nutritional yeast, tamari or liquid coconut aminos, and lemon juice and simmer for 5 minutes.

7. Serve immediately, or let cool and store in an airtight container in the fridge for up to 4 days or in the freezer for up to 1 month.

## Mixed Broth & Ginger Soup Ⓜ

Makes 2 servings

### INGREDIENTS

1 tablespoon extra virgin
  coconut oil
2 cups chopped chives
1-inch knob ginger, peeled
  and grated
Pinch asafetida‡ (aka hing;
  see tip)
2 stalks lemongrass,
  chopped very fine, or 1
  teaspoon lemongrass
  powder
1 (9-ounce) can additive-
  free coconut milk, plus
  more for serving
2 cups Gut-Friendly Mixed
  Broth (page 186 or
  store-bought)
Grated zest and juice of 1
  lemon, plus extra lemon
  juice for serving
2 tablespoons liquid
  coconut aminos
1 tablespoon red wine
  vinegar
Celtic sea salt and freshly
  cracked black pepper,
  to taste

### STEPS

1. In a medium saucepan, melt the oil over medium heat.

2. Add the chives, ginger, asafetida, and lemongrass and cook, stirring frequently, for 3 minutes, or until soft.

3. Pour in the coconut milk and broth and stir.

4. Bring to a boil, then reduce the heat to low and simmer for 5 minutes.

5. Add the lemon zest and juice, liquid aminos, and red wine vinegar.

6. Season to taste with salt and pepper, and serve with extra lemon juice and coconut milk, if desired.

**GutSMART Tip:** *For the pinch asafetida, I recommend Naturevibe Botanicals Organic Asafetida Powder. And if you're looking for a good store-bought mixed broth brand, my favorite is Bonafide Frontier Blend Bone Broth.*

‡ Asafetida (also known as hing) is a seasoning common in South Indian cuisine. When raw, it has a pungent, sulfurous odor, but it smells like leek when cooked. Asafetida is used in India as a digestive aid, since it is known to help reduce gassiness.

## 📷 Beef Pho with Zucchini Noodles ⓜ

Makes 4 servings

### INGREDIENTS

1 tablespoon extra virgin coconut oil

4 ounces beef bones (shin, knuckles, marrow, and gelatinous cuts)

6 star anise pods

2 cinnamon sticks

3 cardamom pods

2 teaspoons coriander seeds

2 teaspoons fennel seeds

8 cups filtered water, or more as needed

2 tablespoons apple cider vinegar

Sea salt and freshly ground black pepper, to taste

½ leek, white part only, thinly sliced

3-inch knob fresh ginger, peeled and chopped

1 tablespoon wheat-free tamari or liquid coconut aminos for soy-free

1 pound grass-fed beef chuck shoulder, thinly sliced

2 zucchinis, spiralized

1 large handful mixed fresh herbs, such as basil, mint, and cilantro

1 handful bean sprouts

2 limes, cut into wedges

### STEPS

1. Preheat the oven to 400°F.

2. Melt the coconut oil in a medium glass or ceramic casserole dish over medium heat.

3. Add the bones and stir to coat. Cover the casserole dish and transfer to the oven.

4. Roast for 30 minutes, or until the bones are browned.

5. Meanwhile, in a small skillet, toast the star anise, cinnamon, cardamom, coriander, and fennel over medium heat for 2 minutes, or until fragrant.

6. After the bones have roasted for 30 minutes, add the toasted spices to the casserole dish, along with the filtered water and apple cider vinegar. Season with salt and pepper.

7. Bring to a boil on the stovetop, then reduce the heat to the lowest setting and simmer, uncovered, for 1½ hours, adding a little more filtered water from time to time, if necessary.

8. Using tongs, carefully remove and discard the bones.

9. Allow the broth to cool, then refrigerate until the fat congeals on top (approximately 1 hour). Scrape off the fat (keep it for cooking with).

10. Add a bit of the fat to the same small skillet and lightly cook the leek and ginger over medium heat, stirring frequently, until softened, about 5 minutes.

11. Transfer the leek and ginger mixture to the casserole dish, add the tamari or coconut aminos and beef, and bring to a boil. Reduce the heat to low and cook until the beef is tender, about 45 minutes.

12. To serve, divide the zucchini noodles into bowls. Add some beef to each bowl, then pour in the boiling broth. Top each serving with the herbs and bean sprouts. Serve with lime wedges.

## Leek & Coconut Soup Ⓜ Ⓜ
Makes 2 servings

### INGREDIENTS

1 tablespoon extra virgin coconut oil
1 scallion, green part only, roughly chopped
1 teaspoon fennel seeds
½ leek, white part only, thinly sliced
1 medium parsnip, peeled and diced*
2¾ cups watercress or arugula, plus more for garnish
1 (9-ounce) can additive-free coconut milk
1½ cups vegetable broth (page 183 or store-bought)
1 teaspoon grated lemon zest
1 tablespoon lemon juice
Celtic sea salt and freshly cracked black pepper, to taste
½ teaspoon dulse, kelp, or seaweed flakes

*Adapt It: If you are in the Mild category, you can choose to substitute turnip for the parsnip.

### STEPS

1. Melt the coconut oil in a medium saucepan over medium heat.

2. Add the scallion and fennel seeds and cook, stirring frequently, for 3 to 4 minutes, until fragrant.

3. Add the leek, parsnip, watercress, coconut milk, and broth and bring to a boil.

4. Reduce the heat to low, add the lemon zest and juice, cover, and simmer for 20 minutes.

5. Remove from the heat and allow to cool slightly, then puree in a blender until smooth.

6. Season to taste, and reheat if necessary. Garnish with extra watercress and dulse, kelp, or seaweed flakes and serve.

## Gut-Balancing Veggie Stew ⓜ

Makes 2 to 3 servings

### INGREDIENTS

1 tablespoon extra virgin olive oil or grass-fed ghee

1 scallion, green part only, finely chopped

Pinch asafetida (hing; see tip on page 191)

1 zucchini, diced

1 large red bell pepper, seeded and diced

1 small eggplant, diced

½ cup chopped broccoli (can include stem pieces if well tolerated)

1 tablespoon dried Italian herb seasoning

1 tablespoon ground turmeric or finely grated fresh turmeric

1 (14-ounce) can coconut cream

Chopped fresh cilantro, for garnish

### STEPS

1. Heat the oil in a medium skillet over medium heat.

2. Add the scallion and asafetida and cook, stirring frequently, for 2 to 3 minutes, until softened.

3. Add the zucchini, bell pepper, eggplant, broccoli, Italian herbs, turmeric, and coconut cream and stir to combine.

4. Reduce the heat to low, cover, and cook for 25 minutes, or until the vegetables are tender.

5. Garnish with fresh cilantro and serve.

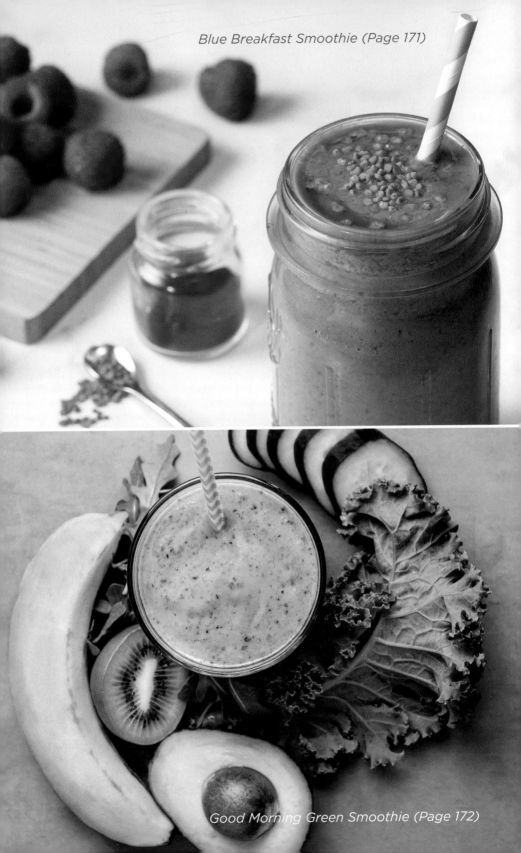

*Blue Breakfast Smoothie (Page 171)*

*Good Morning Green Smoothie (Page 172)*

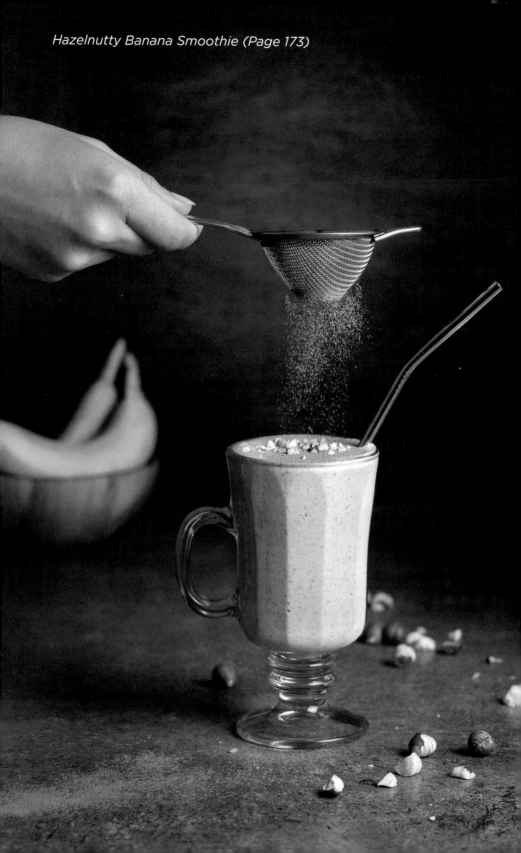

*Hazelnutty Banana Smoothie (Page 173)*

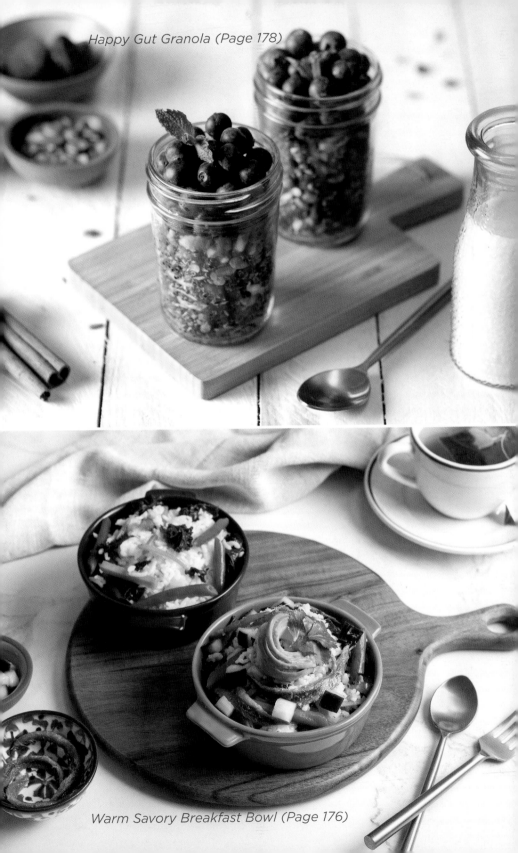

Happy Gut Granola (Page 178)

Warm Savory Breakfast Bowl (Page 176)

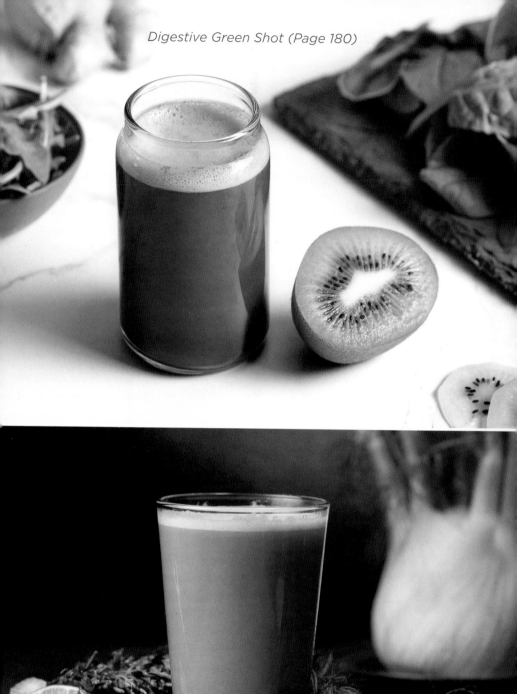

*Digestive Green Shot (Page 180)*

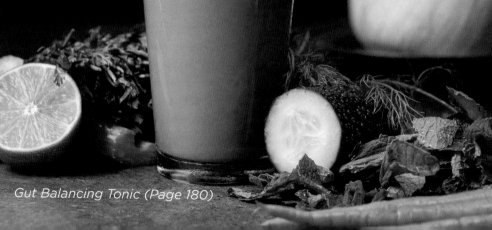

*Gut Balancing Tonic (Page 180)*

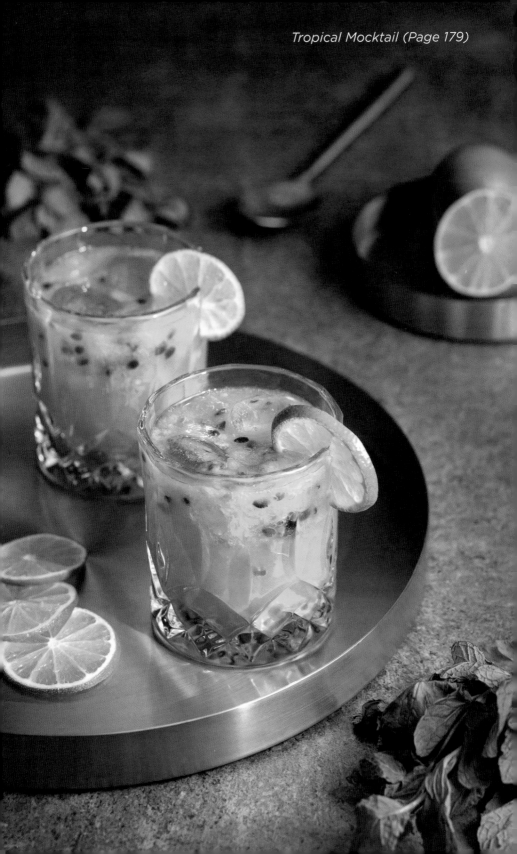

*Tropical Mocktail (Page 179)*

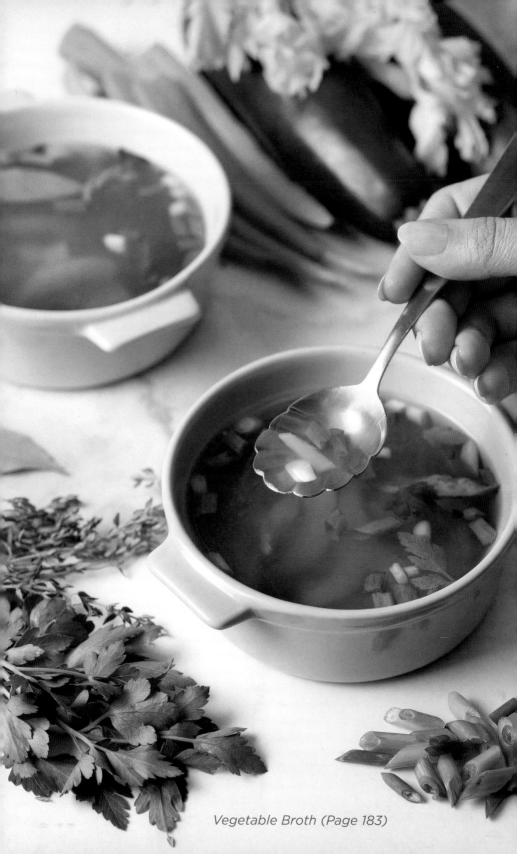

*Vegetable Broth (Page 183)*

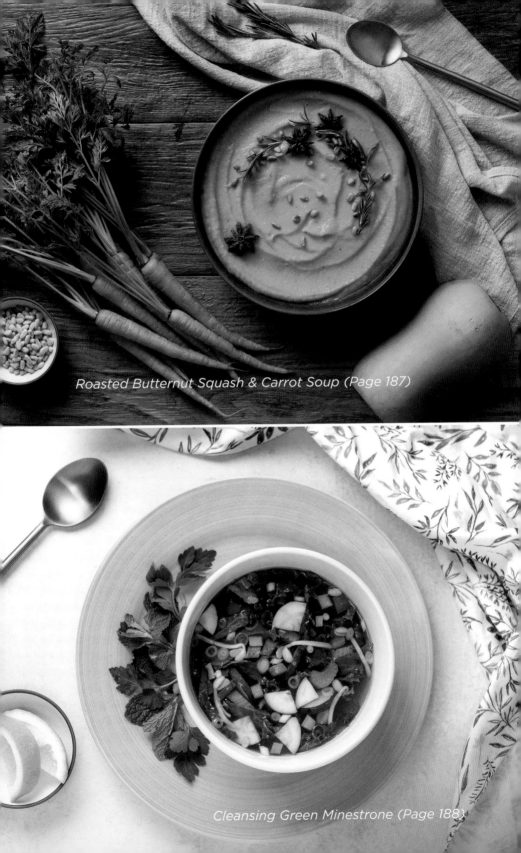

Roasted Butternut Squash & Carrot Soup (Page 187)

Cleansing Green Minestrone (Page 188)

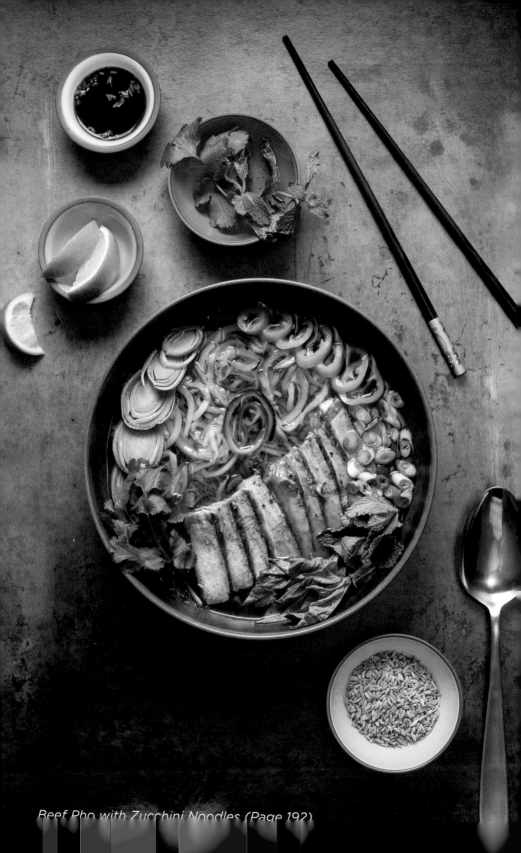

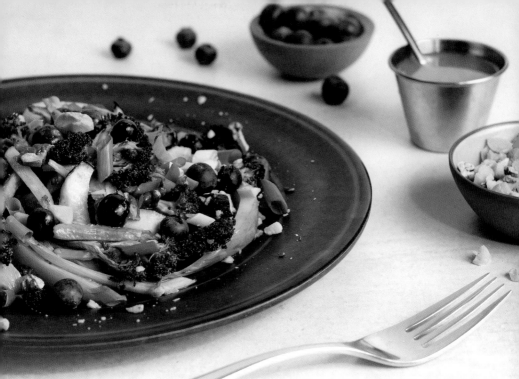

*Baked Super Green & Berry Salad with Macadamia Dressing (Page 196)*

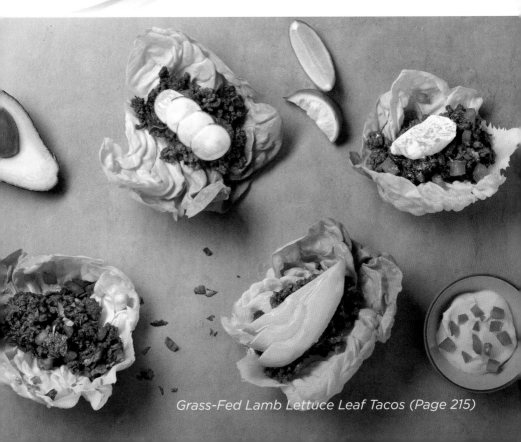

*Grass-Fed Lamb Lettuce Leaf Tacos (Page 215)*

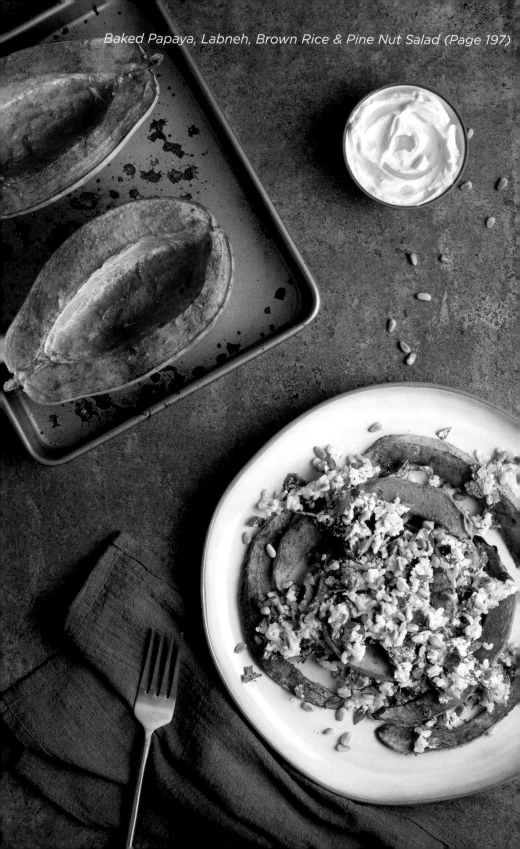

Baked Papaya, Labneh, Brown Rice & Pine Nut Salad (Page 197)

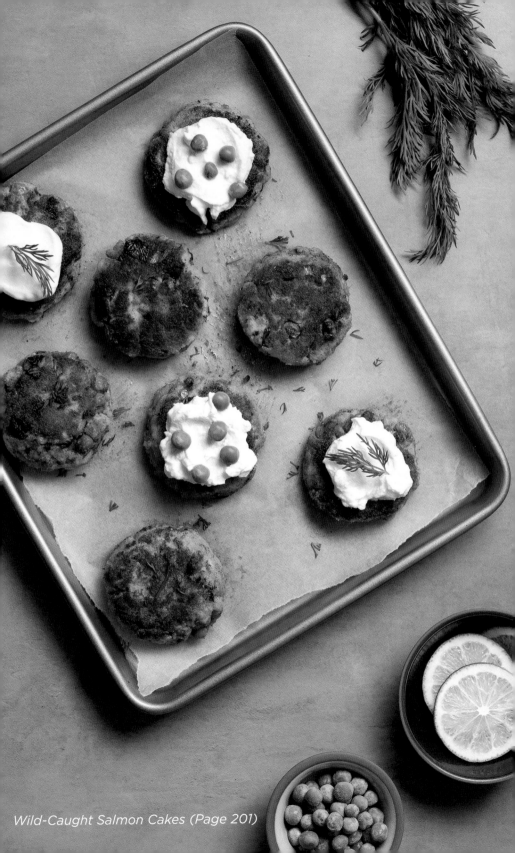

*Wild-Caught Salmon Cakes (Page 201)*

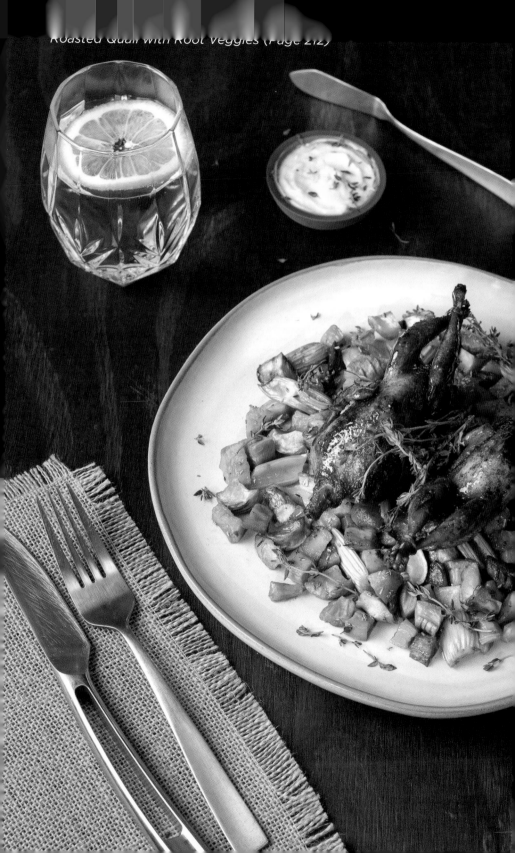

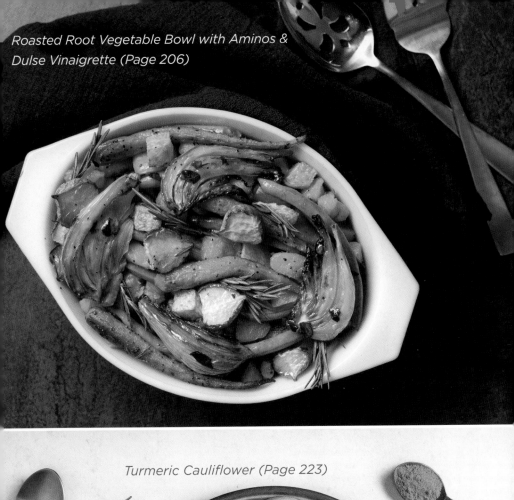

Roasted Root Vegetable Bowl with Aminos &
Dulse Vinaigrette (Page 206)

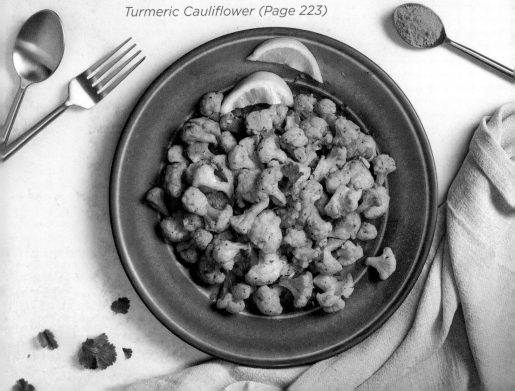

Turmeric Cauliflower (Page 223)

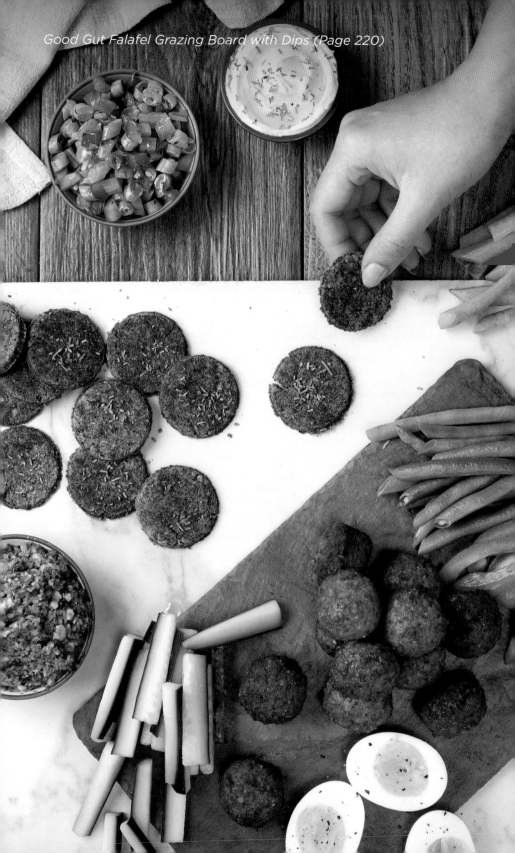

Good Gut Falafel Grazing Board with Dips (Page 220)

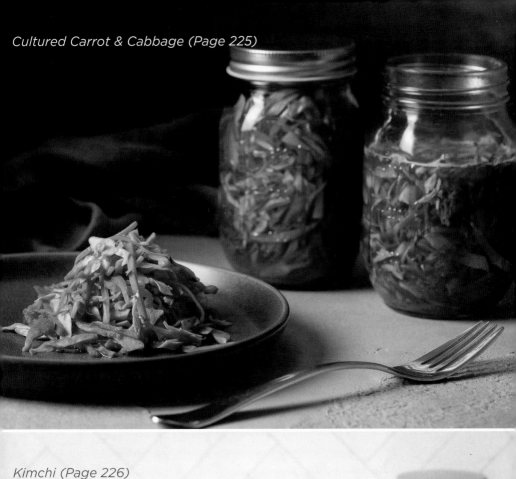
*Cultured Carrot & Cabbage (Page 225)*

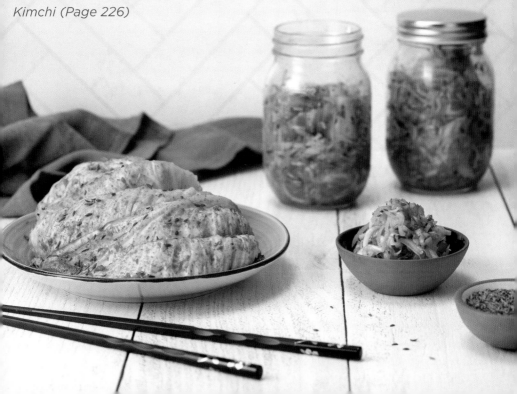
*Kimchi (Page 226)*

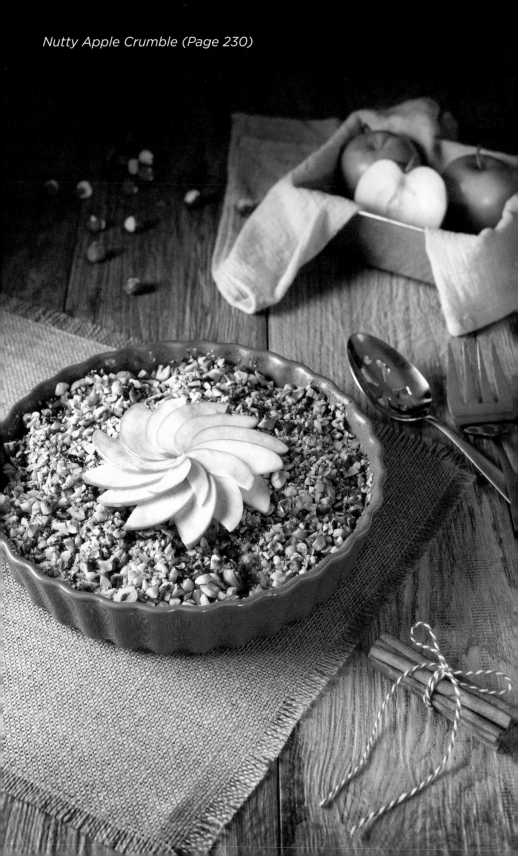

*Nutty Apple Crumble (Page 230)*

# SAVORY SALADS

*What I love most about salads is the explosion of colors and flavors that can be combined on one plate. These savory salads can serve as a main or side dish. One of my favorites is the Baked Papaya, Labneh, Brown Rice & Pine Nut Salad (see color insert).*

## Crunchy Kaleslaw with Lime & Sesame Dressing Ⓢ
Makes 3 to 4 servings

### INGREDIENTS

**Slaw**

1 bunch kale, stemmed
   and chopped
6 carrots, peeled and
   shredded
¼ red cabbage, shredded
1 avocado, pitted, peeled,
   and diced
1 bunch scallions, green
   parts only, chopped

**Dressing**

1 tablespoon toasted
   sesame seeds
3 tablespoons extra virgin
   olive oil
2 tablespoons lime juice
1 tablespoon wheat-free
   tamari or liquid coconut
   aminos for soy-free
½ teaspoon stevia
   (optional)

### STEPS

1. Combine all the slaw ingredients in a large bowl.

2. Combine all the dressing ingredients in a small jar or cup and shake or whisk to combine.

3. Add the dressing to the slaw and toss well to coat. Serve immediately.

## 📷 Baked Super Green & Berry Salad with Macadamia Dressing Ⓢ Ⓜ 🔗

Makes 2 servings

### INGREDIENTS

**Salad**

1 cup chopped broccoli
    florets*
1 large zucchini, chopped
10 green beans, sliced
½ fennel bulb, chopped
1 scallion, green part only,
    thinly sliced
Sea salt and freshly
    ground pepper, to taste
2 tablespoons extra virgin
    olive oil
2 tablespoons chopped
    pecans
20 macadamias, crushed
¼ cup blueberries

**Dressing**

¼ cup macadamia oil
1 tablespoon lemon juice*
1 tablespoon honey
1 teaspoon sugar-free,
    garlic-free stone-
    ground mustard

*Adapt It: To adapt this
salad for the Moderate
category, substitute 1
tablespoon apple cider
vinegar for the lemon juice
and increase the chopped
broccoli to 2 cups.*

### STEPS

1. Preheat the oven to 400°F. Line a rimmed baking sheet with parchment paper.

2. Combine the broccoli, zucchini, green beans, fennel, and scallion in a large bowl and season with salt and pepper.

3. Drizzle the olive oil over the vegetables, and rub it in with your hands until the vegetables are well coated.

4. Spread out the vegetables on the prepared baking sheet and roast for 35 to 45 minutes, until all the vegetables are caramelized, checking now and then and removing any vegetables that are done.

5. Set the vegetables aside to cool slightly.

6. Meanwhile, combine all the dressing ingredients in a small jar and shake well.

7. Transfer the vegetables to a large bowl. Pour the dressing over the vegetables and gently toss.

8. Add the pecans, macadamias, and blueberries and serve.

SAVORY SALADS

# Baked Papaya, Labneh, Brown Rice & Pine Nut Salad Ⓜ ✐

Makes 1 or 2 servings

## INGREDIENTS

1 papaya, halved and seeded
1 teaspoon sweet paprika
Grated zest and juice of 1 lime
1½ cups cooked brown rice
1¼ cups chopped fresh parsley
3 tablespoons labneh or plain coconut yogurt for dairy-free
2 tablespoons extra virgin olive oil
Sea salt and freshly ground black pepper, to taste
3 tablespoons pine nuts, toasted
1 tablespoon sacha inchi oil,‡ flaxseed oil, or more olive oil

## STEPS

1. Preheat the oven to 350°F. Line a rimmed baking sheet with parchment paper.

2. Place the papaya halves on the prepared baking sheet. Sprinkle with the paprika and lime zest and drizzle with the lime juice. Bake for about 15 minutes, until the papaya is lightly colored. Set aside to cool slightly.

3. On a platter, toss together the brown rice, parsley, labneh or coconut yogurt, and olive oil and season with salt and pepper.

4. Cut the papaya lengthwise into long strips, then crosswise into bite-size cubes.

5. Add the papaya to the rice mixture. Scatter the pine nuts over the top and add a drizzle of sacha inchi oil. Serve.

*GutSMART Tip:* Instead of labneh or coconut yogurt, you can use ½ cup crumbled tempeh. In a small skillet, heat 1 tablespoon olive oil over medium heat. Panfry ½ cup crumbled tempeh for a few minutes, until crispy, before adding to the rice mixture.

‡ **Sacha inchi**, sometimes referred to as the "mountain peanut" or "Inca nut," because it was consumed by the indigenous people of Peru, contains a large edible seed that is rich in protein, fiber, micronutrients, and heart-healthy fats. The seeds can be roasted and eaten or pressed into an oil, as is called for in this recipe.

## Spiced Roast Butternut Squash & Leftover Lamb Salad Ⓜ 🖐

Makes 2 servings

### INGREDIENTS

**Dressing**

2 tablespoons tahini
Juice of ½ lemon
1 tablespoon honey
Pinch sea salt and freshly
  cracked pepper
2–3 tablespoons warm
  water

**Salad**

1 cup cherry tomatoes
3 tablespoons garlic-
  infused olive oil, divided
  in thirds
Pinch or two fresh thyme
  leaves
1 butternut squash, halved,
  seeded, and cut into
  small wedges
½ teaspoon ground cumin
½ teaspoon ground
  coriander
¼ teaspoon ground
  cinnamon
1 tablespoon grated fresh
  ginger
Sea salt and freshly
  cracked black pepper,
  to taste
8 ounces lamb loin or
  leftover Sunday Braised
  Lamb on Butternut
  Squash Mash (page
  216)
3 large handfuls mixed
  leaf lettuce
1 cup cooked or thawed
  frozen peas
½ cup chopped fresh
  buffalo mozzarella
1 handful fresh basil leaves

### STEPS

1. Preheat the oven to 400°F.

2. To make the dressing, combine the tahini,
   lemon juice, honey, and salt and pepper in a
   small jar or cup. Whisk thoroughly, gradually
   adding a little warm water until the dressing is
   smooth, thick, and creamy. Set aside.

3. To make the salad, scatter the tomatoes on
   one side of a rimmed baking sheet, drizzle with
   1 tablespoon of the oil, and sprinkle with the
   thyme leaves.

4. In a bowl, toss the squash wedges with the
   cumin, coriander, cinnamon, and ginger until
   coated. Place the squash on the other side of the
   baking sheet, drizzle with another 1 tablespoon
   olive oil, and season with salt and pepper.

5. Roast for 20 minutes, or until the tomato skins
   are beginning to burst. Transfer the tomatoes
   to a plate and return the baking sheet to the
   oven. Continue roasting the squash wedges for
   another 10 minutes, until golden and crispy.

6. Meanwhile, if using uncooked lamb, season
   it with salt and pepper. Heat the remaining 1
   tablespoon oil in a skillet over medium heat.
   Cook the lamb loin for 3 minutes on each side;
   it should still be pink in the center. Let it rest
   for a few minutes, then cut into ¼-inch slices.
   If using leftover sliced lamb, heat it briefly in a
   skillet until warmed through.

7. To arrange the salad, make a bed of mixed salad leaves, and top with the warm squash, lamb, tomatoes, and peas. Drizzle the tahini dressing generously over the top. Garnish with fresh mozzarella and basil leaves, and serve warm.

## Goat Cheese, Sprouted Pumpkin Seed & Asparagus Salad Ⓜ
Makes 2 servings

### INGREDIENTS

3 tablespoons olive oil, divided in thirds
3 tablespoons sprouted pumpkin seeds
1 teaspoon smoked paprika
4 asparagus spears, trimmed and cut into 1-inch pieces
1 teaspoon lemon juice
1 teaspoon maple syrup
½ teaspoon coriander seeds (optional)
Sea salt and freshly cracked pepper, to taste
3 cups mixed greens, such as watercress, baby spinach, arugula, and endive
¼ cup goat cheese or vegan feta cheese, crumbled

### STEPS

1. Heat 1 tablespoon of the olive oil in a medium skillet over a low heat. Add the sprouted pumpkin seeds and sprinkle with the smoked paprika. Cook, stirring constantly, until golden, 2 to 5 minutes. Transfer the seeds to a plate and set aside.

2. Heat another 1 tablespoon olive oil in the same skillet over low heat. Add the asparagus and cook for 5 minutes, or until softened. Remove from the heat.

3. In a small bowl or cup, whisk together the remaining 1 tablespoon olive oil, the lemon juice, maple syrup, coriander seeds (if using), salt, and pepper.

4. Toss the mixed greens together in a bowl. Add the asparagus and goat cheese, then pour the dressing over and toss gently. Sprinkle the pumpkin seeds on top and serve.

# ENTREES (BEEF, POULTRY, WILD GAME, FISH, VEGAN)

*From stuffed sweet peppers to Wild-Caught Salmon Cakes (see color insert) to colorful vegan dishes (see the Roasted Root Vegetable Bowl with Aminos & Dulse Vinaigrette in color insert), there's something for everyone in these gut-friendly entrees. And for a really special treat, try the Sunday Braised Lamb on Butternut Squash Mash.*

## Stuffed Sweet Peppers with Lamb Ⓢ
Makes 4 servings

### INGREDIENTS

2 tablespoons extra virgin olive oil, divided in half
1 cup sliced scallions, green parts only
12 ounces ground lamb
1 teaspoon sea salt
Freshly ground black pepper
1 teaspoon dried or fresh rosemary
1 teaspoon ground coriander
½ cup chopped English cucumber
1½ cups cooked white rice
1 tablespoon grass-fed ghee or refined coconut oil for dairy-free
2 red bell peppers
2 yellow bell peppers
Handful chopped fresh parsley, for garnish
Nutritional yeast flakes, for garnish
1 tablespoon pine nuts, toasted, for garnish (optional)

### STEPS

1. Preheat the oven to 400°F.

2. Heat 1 tablespoon of the oil in a large skillet over medium heat. Add the scallions and cook for 2 to 5 minutes, until softened.

3. Add the lamb, season with the salt and pepper, and cook, stirring frequently, for 5 minutes, or until the lamb is cooked through.

4. Stir in the rosemary, coriander, cucumber, rice, and ghee or coconut oil. Turn the heat down and simmer for 5 minutes.

5. Slice the tops off the peppers and scoop out the seeds and ribs. Stand the peppers upright in a baking dish and drizzle with the remaining 1 tablespoon oil. Spoon some of the lamb mixture into each pepper.

6. Bake until the peppers are tender, about 35 minutes. Garnish with parsley, nutritional yeast flakes, and pine nuts (if using) before serving.

## Wild-Caught Salmon Cakes **S**

Makes 4

### INGREDIENTS

8 ounces fresh or canned
  wild-caught salmon
½ cup thawed frozen peas
1 cup sliced scallions,
  green parts only
2 tablespoons chopped
  fresh dill
1 tablespoon chopped
  fresh cilantro, plus more
  for garnish
1 tablespoon honey
1 tablespoon lime juice
2 teaspoons sugar-free,
  garlic-free stone-
  ground mustard
1 teaspoon coconut milk
  or water (optional)
Celtic sea salt and freshly
  ground black pepper,
  to taste
2 tablespoons coconut
  flour
2 teaspoons coconut oil
Lime wedges, for serving

### STEPS

1. Drain the salmon (if canned) and place it in a medium bowl. Remove the bones if needed, then mash the flesh with a fork.

2. Add the peas, scallions, dill, cilantro, honey, lime juice, mustard, and coconut milk (if needed for moisture). Season with salt and pepper and mix well.

3. Roll the mixture into a big ball, then cover and chill in the freezer for 30 minutes.

4. Divide the chilled mixture into four equal portions. Shape each portion into a patty. Put the coconut flour on a plate and dust each patty on both sides in the flour.

5. Heat the oil in a medium skillet over medium heat. Add the salmon cakes and cook for 7 to 10 minutes on each side, until golden brown. Serve warm, with lime wedges for squeezing.

## Lemongrass Poached Chicken with Green Beans **S**

Makes 4 servings

### INGREDIENTS

8 cups filtered water
4 lemongrass tea bags
1 lemongrass stalk, pale part only
½ teaspoon fennel seeds
1 tablespoon finely grated lime zest
3–4 makrut lime leaves or ½ teaspoon grated lime zest
4 small organic boneless, skinless chicken breasts
1 teaspoon grass-fed ghee or refined coconut oil for dairy-free
1 scallion, green part only, thinly sliced
1 tablespoon lime juice, plus for serving
1 tablespoon wheat-free tamari or liquid coconut aminos for soy-free
2 cups green beans, trimmed and cut into 1-inch pieces
Sea salt and freshly ground black pepper, to taste
1 tablespoon sesame seeds, toasted

### STEPS

1. In a medium saucepan, combine the water, tea bags, lemongrass, fennel seeds, lime zest, and lime leaves. Bring to a boil, then cover, turn off the heat, and leave for 10 minutes to steep.

2. Strain the tea, then return the liquid to the saucepan and bring to a simmer.

3. Add the chicken breasts and simmer for 9 to 12 minutes, until they are cooked through and no longer pink inside when tested with a knife.

4. Remove the chicken from the liquid, reserving the liquid, and slice into long, thin pieces; set aside.

5. Melt the ghee or coconut oil in a medium skillet over medium heat. Add the scallion and stir-fry for 1 to 2 minutes. Add the lime juice, tamari or coconut aminos, and ⅔ cup of the reserved tea and stir to combine. Add the green beans and cook for 5 to 6 minutes, until the beans start to soften.

6. Transfer the chicken to a serving plate, season with salt and pepper, add a squeeze of lime, then top with the green beans and cooking liquid. Sprinkle over the sesame seeds and serve.

**GutSMART Tip:** *This is a great dish to prepare ahead of time and have as a snack or serve as an appetizer at a gathering.*

## Seared Tuna with Squash Puree & Herbs ⑤

Makes 2 servings

### INGREDIENTS

**Squash Puree**

½ cup peeled and cubed kabocha or butternut squash

1 tablespoon almond milk (page 172 or store-bought) or hemp milk for nut-free

2 teaspoons extra virgin coconut oil

1 teaspoon sugar-free, garlic-free stone-ground mustard

Pink Himalayan or Celtic sea salt

**Tuna**

1 tablespoon extra virgin olive oil, plus more for brushing and drizzling

½ cup thinly sliced scallions, green parts only

2 wild-caught tuna steaks

Sea salt and freshly ground black pepper, to taste

½ cup green peas, cooked or thawed frozen

Large handful fresh mint or cilantro leaves

2 tablespoons sesame seeds, toasted

### STEPS

1. Bring a small saucepan of water to a boil, then add the squash cubes and cook until just tender. Drain. Transfer to a blender and blend, gradually adding the almond milk until smooth. Add the coconut oil and mustard and blend. Season with a pinch of salt.

2. Heat the olive oil in a medium skillet over medium heat. Sauté the scallions for a few minutes until golden, then transfer to a small bowl.

3. Brush the tuna steaks with more olive oil and season with salt and pepper. Add them to the skillet and cook for 2 to 3 minutes on each side, or until cooked to your liking.

4. Serve the tuna steaks on a bed of squash puree, drizzled with a little olive oil.

5. Garnish with the sautéed scallions, and top with the peas, herbs, and sesame seeds.

**GutSMART Tip:** *You can also serve the tuna with white rice, but limit to ½ cup per person in the Severe category.*

## Ground Beef with Peas Indian Style ⑤

Makes 4 servings

**INGREDIENTS**

2 tablespoons grass-fed ghee or refined coconut oil for dairy-free

2 scallions, green parts only, sliced

¼ teaspoon asafetida or ground coriander

1 teaspoon ground cardamom

1 small star anise pod

2 whole cloves

½ teaspoon Himalayan salt, plus more to taste

1 pound ground beef

½ cup coconut milk, or more if desired

1 cup frozen baby peas

Freshly cracked black pepper, to taste

Filtered water (optional)

Handful fresh cilantro, for serving

⅔ cup whole walnuts, chopped, for serving (optional)

2 cups cooked rice, for serving

**STEPS**

1. Heat the ghee or coconut oil in a wok or large skillet over medium heat. Add the scallions and cook for 3 minutes, or until soft.

2. Add the asafetida, cardamom, star anise, cloves, and salt and stir for a few seconds.

3. Add the ground beef and cook, stirring frequently to break up the meat as it cooks, until it turns from pink to brown, 10 to 15 minutes.

4. Stir in the coconut milk and peas, then reduce the heat to low, cover, and cook for 15 minutes.

5. Season with salt and pepper. If you prefer a moister dish, add more coconut milk.

6. Sprinkle with cilantro and chopped walnuts and serve with white rice.

## Grass-Fed Lamb with Broccoli Mash Ⓢ
Makes 2 to 3 servings

### INGREDIENTS

**Broccoli Mash**

1 large head broccoli,
 roughly chopped
1 tablespoon grass-fed
 ghee or refined coconut
 oil for dairy-free
2 scallions, green parts
 only, chopped
Celtic sea salt and freshly
 cracked black pepper,
 to taste

**Lamb Loin**

1 (9-ounce) grass-fed
 lamb loin
1 tablespoon chopped
 fresh or dried rosemary
Sea salt and freshly
 cracked black pepper,
 to taste
1 tablespoon coconut oil
1 red bell pepper, seeded
 and thinly sliced
 lengthwise

**Garnish**

2 cups microgreens
1 cup watercress
1 tablespoon dulse or
 seaweed flakes

### STEPS

1. Bring a large saucepan of water to a boil, then add the broccoli and cook for 5 to 6 minutes, until al dente. Drain and set aside.

2. Melt the ghee or coconut oil in the same saucepan over medium heat. Add the scallions and cook, stirring frequently, for 2 minutes, or until soft.

3. Puree the broccoli and scallions in a food processor until smooth or to the desired consistency, adding a touch more ghee if needed, and season to taste.

4. Season the lamb with the rosemary and salt and pepper.

5. Melt the coconut oil in a large skillet over medium heat. Add the bell pepper and cook for 2 minutes, or until softened.

6. Add the lamb and cook for 3 minutes on each side (it should still be pink in the center). Transfer to a cutting board and let it rest for about 5 minutes, then cut into ¼-inch slices.

7. Serve the lamb with the bell pepper and broccoli mash. Garnish with the microgreens and watercress and sprinkle the dulse flakes over the top.

**GutSMART Tip:** *For best flavor, season room-temperature lamb one hour before cooking.*

## 📷 Roasted Root Vegetable Bowl with Aminos & Dulse Vinaigrette ⑤

Makes 3 to 4 servings

### INGREDIENTS

**Vegetable Bowl**

1 cup peeled and cubed
   butternut squash
2 fennel bulbs, peeled and
   quartered lengthwise
2 large rutabagas, peeled
   and cut into cubes
1 cup baby carrots,
   trimmed
1 cup trimmed and halved
   radishes
¼ cup extra virgin olive oil
1 tablespoon fennel seeds
1 tablespoon fresh or dried
   rosemary
2 cups trimmed and
   halved green beans

**Aminos and Dulse
   Vinaigrette**

¼ cup olive oil
¼ cup lemon juice
Pinch Celtic sea salt
1 tablespoon sugar-free,
   garlic-free stone-
   ground mustard
2 teaspoons clover honey
2 teaspoons liquid
   coconut aminos
1 teaspoon dulse flakes

### STEPS

1. Preheat the oven to 400°F. Line a large roasting pan with parchment paper.

2. Spread out the butternut squash, fennel, rutabagas, carrots, and radishes in a single layer in the prepared baking pan. Drizzle with the olive oil, ensuring that everything is covered. Sprinkle on the fennel seeds and rosemary.

3. Roast for 25 minutes, turning the vegetables once and removing any that have cooked through.

4. Add the green beans and roast for another 10 minutes, or until all the vegetables are golden. (The rutabagas will take 35 to 40 minutes total.)

5. Meanwhile, combine all the vinaigrette ingredients in a small bowl or jar and whisk or shake to mix well.

6. Serve the roasted vegetables with the vinaigrette drizzled on top.

**GutSMART Tip:** *You can also serve this with white rice, but limit to ½ cup per person if in the Severe category.*

## Aromatic Chicken Curry Ⓢ Ⓜ Ⓜ

Makes 2 to 3 servings

### INGREDIENTS

**Chicken**

2 teaspoons ground coriander

1 teaspoon ground cardamom

1 teaspoon fennel seed

2 tablespoons lemon juice

1½ pounds organic boneless, skinless chicken thighs, cut in half

1 tablespoon coconut oil

1 cup sliced scallions, green parts only

¼ cup diced fennel bulb

1 cup additive-free coconut milk

2 makrut lime leaves, thinly sliced, or ¼ teaspoon grated lime zest

2 cardamom pods

**Cauliflower Rice**

¼ cup coconut oil

1 head cauliflower, riced (you can do this in a food processor or high-speed blender)

Handful fresh cilantro leaves, roughly chopped

Sea salt and freshly ground black pepper, to taste

*\*Adapt It: Adapt this recipe for Moderate category by adding 1 teaspoon curry powder, 1 teaspoon ground ginger, 1 teaspoon ground turmeric, and 1 teaspoon ground cumin. And when your GutSMART score is Mild, you can also heat this up a bit by adding some chili flakes to taste.*

### STEPS

1. In a large bowl, whisk together the coriander, cardamom, fennel seed, and lemon juice. Add the chicken pieces, coat well, cover, and marinate in the fridge for at least 1 hour.

2. Heat the coconut oil in a large skillet over medium heat. Add the scallions and fennel and cook, stirring, for 2 to 3 minutes, until softened.

3. Add the chicken and brown for 5 to 7 minutes on each side.

4. Add the coconut milk, lime leaves, and cardamom pods and simmer for 15 minutes, or until the chicken is tender.

5. Meanwhile, to make the cauliflower rice, melt the oil in another large skillet over medium heat. Add the cauliflower and most of the cilantro (save some for garnish) and season with salt and pepper. Cook for 8 to 10 minutes, until soft.

6. Spoon the cauliflower rice into bowls, top with the chicken, and garnish with the reserved cilantro.

## Snow Pea, Zucchini & Coconut Casserole Ⓢ

Makes 2 to 3 servings

### INGREDIENTS

1 teaspoon grass-fed ghee
  or refined coconut oil
  for dairy-free
1 scallion, chopped
1 teaspoon ground
  coriander
1 teaspoon ground
  cardamom
1 star anise pod, broken up
1 teaspoon ground sage
½ teaspoon asafetida
  or additional ground
  coriander
1 makrut lime leaf, thinly
  sliced
4 zucchinis, cut into
  batons (size of your
  little finger)
1 cup vegetable
  broth (page 183 or
  store-bought)
⅓ cup additive-free
  coconut milk
1 tablespoon coconut flour
1 teaspoon grated lime
  zest
1 tablespoon lime juice
Celtic sea salt and freshly
  ground black pepper,
  to taste
10 snow pea pods, cut in
  half crosswise
Filtered water, as needed
2 teaspoons alfalfa or
  clover honey
1½ cups cooked white rice,
  for serving
Fresh cilantro leaves, for
  garnish

### STEPS

1. Heat the ghee or coconut oil in a medium saucepan over low heat. Add the scallion, coriander, cardamom, star anise, sage, asafetida, and lime leaf and cook, stirring, for 2 to 3 minutes.

2. Add the zucchinis and cook for 2 minutes.

3. Add the vegetable broth, coconut milk, coconut flour, and lime zest and juice, then season with salt and pepper and stir to integrate the coconut flour.

4. Add the snow peas and bring to a gentle boil, then reduce the heat to medium-low and simmer for 5 minutes, or until the zucchini is tender and the sauce has thickened.

5. Stir in the honey and season to taste.

6. Serve over white rice, topped with cilantro leaves.

## Spanish Jamon Serrano Frittata Ⓜ ⓘ

Makes 4 to 5 servings

### INGREDIENTS

9 large pasture-raised eggs

Celtic sea salt and freshly ground pepper, to taste

1 small handful basil leaves, roughly chopped

2 tablespoons extra virgin olive oil

3 scallions, green parts only, chopped

1 red bell pepper, seeded and diced

⅔ cup chopped preservative-free Spanish jamon serrano or preservative-free ham of choice

15 baby spinach leaves

3 kale leaves, stemmed and chopped

2 tablespoons nutritional yeast flakes

### STEPS

1. Preheat the broiler to high heat.

2. Whisk the eggs, salt, and pepper together in a large bowl. Add the basil and stir.

3. Heat the olive oil in a large oven-proof skillet over medium heat. Add the scallions and cook, stirring occasionally, for 2 minutes, or until softened.

4. Add the bell pepper and ham and cook, stirring occasionally, for 3 minutes.

5. Add the spinach and kale and cook for 2 minutes, or until wilted.

6. Pour the egg mixture over the vegetables and cook for 5 to 7 minutes, until just set.

7. Sprinkle on the yeast flakes and place the skillet under the broiler for 3 minutes, or until the top of the frittata is lightly browned.

8. Allow to cool slightly, then slice and serve.

## Bunless Grass-Fed Beef Burger Ⓜ ⓪
Makes 5 servings

### INGREDIENTS

2 radishes, thinly sliced
¼ red cabbage, thinly sliced
2 cups chopped fresh flat-leaf parsley
3 tablespoons extra virgin olive oil, divided (2 tablespoons + 1 tablespoon)
Juice of 1 lemon
1 tablespoon avocado oil mayonnaise
Sea salt and freshly ground black pepper, to taste
1 pound ground grass-fed beef
¼ leek, white part only, sliced
1 large pasture-raised egg, lightly beaten
1 teaspoon dried sage
Pinch paprika (optional)
10 romaine lettuce leaves
2 baby beets or 1 medium beet, thinly sliced
Crispy Sweet Potato Fries (page 219), for serving

### STEPS

1. In a large bowl, combine the radishes, cabbage, parsley, 2 tablespoons of the olive oil, the lemon juice, mayo, salt, and pepper. Toss to coat evenly. Set aside.

2. In another large bowl, combine the beef, leek, egg, sage, paprika (if using), salt, and pepper. Divide the mixture into 5 equal portions, then form into patties.

3. Heat the remaining 1 tablespoon oil in a large skillet over medium heat.

4. Add the patties and cook for 4 minutes, then flip and cook for an additional 3 minutes, or until cooked through or desired doneness.

5. Place each patty on a lettuce leaf. Add some of the cabbage mixture and beet slices, then top with another lettuce leaf.

6. Serve with sweet potato fries.

**GutSMART Tip:** *For a leaner, wild option, substitute ground bison for the ground beef and cook the patties for 4 minutes on the first side and about 2 minutes on the other.*

## Flaxseed-Crusted Wild-Caught Salmon Ⓜ ⓪

Makes 2 servings

### INGREDIENTS

1 large pasture-raised egg
  white
1 tablespoon water
⅓ cup plus 2 tablespoons
  ground flaxseeds
2 teaspoons dried Italian
  herb seasoning or
  herbes de Provence
2 (5-ounce) skin-on, wild-
  caught salmon fillets
Celtic sea salt and freshly
  ground black pepper,
  to taste
2 tablespoons extra virgin
  olive oil
2 cups crunchy mixed
  green lettuce leaves
1 cup cooked brown rice
2 lime wedges

### STEPS

1.  Preheat the oven to 400°F. Line a rimmed
    baking sheet with parchment paper.

2.  In a small bowl, whisk together the egg white
    and water.

3.  In a large, shallow bowl, combine 2 tablespoons
    of the ground flaxseeds and the Italian herbs to
    make a mixture.

4.  Season the salmon fillets with salt and pepper.
    Coat the fillets with the rest of the ground
    flaxseed, brush with the egg white mixture, then
    dip into the flaxseed and herb mixture.

5.  Heat the oil in a large skillet over medium
    heat. Carefully place the salmon fillets in the
    pan, skin side down. Sear for 2 minutes. Using
    a spatula, carefully flip the fillets and cook for
    another 2 to 3 minutes, until well seared.

6.  Transfer the salmon to the prepared baking
    sheet. Bake for 10 minutes.

7.  Serve with the mixed lettuce leaves and brown
    rice and garnish with the lime wedges.

# 📷 Roasted Quail with Root Veggies Ⓜ 🖊

Makes 2 servings

## INGREDIENTS

¼ cup olive oil
1 tablespoon paprika
1 teaspoon onion powder
Celtic sea salt and freshly
   cracked black pepper,
   to taste
2 quails
4 thyme sprigs
1 small sweet potato,
   peeled and diced
1 small celery root, peeled
   and diced
1 parsnip, peeled and
   roughly chopped
½ cup grass-fed ghee,
   melted, divided in half

## STEPS

1.  1. Preheat the oven to 350°F.

2.  Mix the olive oil, paprika, onion powder, a
    pinch of salt, and a few grinds of pepper in a
    large bowl. Add the quails and massage the rub
    all over. Leave to rest in the fridge while you
    prepare the vegetables.

3.  In a roasting pan, make a bed of thyme sprigs,
    sweet potato, celery root, and parsnip. Season
    with salt and pepper. Pour ¼ cup of the ghee
    over the vegetables.

4.  Roast for 20 minutes, turning the vegetables
    occasionally.

5.  Meanwhile, in a large skillet, heat the remaining
    ¼ cup ghee over medium heat. Add the quails
    and brown for 2 to 3 minutes per side.

6.  Carefully place the quails on top of the
    vegetables. Pour the ghee from the skillet on
    top.

7.  Return the roasting pan to the oven and roast
    for 25 to 30 minutes, until the quails are cooked
    through.

8.  Remove the roasting dish from oven and place
    directly on the table for serving. Top with finely
    ground Celtic sea salt and a pinch of freshly
    cracked black pepper.

## Fish & Lime Curry Ⓜ Ⓜ

Makes 4 servings

### INGREDIENTS

**Lime Curry Paste**

1 cup chopped fresh
  chives
½-inch knob ginger,
  peeled and grated
2 lemongrass stalks, white
  parts only, very finely
  chopped
1½ tablespoons honey
1 tablespoon extra virgin
  olive oil*
1 tablespoon curry powder
1 teaspoon ground
  turmeric
1 teaspoon grated lime
  zest
1 teaspoon extra virgin
  coconut oil

**Fish and Rice**

1 (13.5-ounce) can
  additive-free coconut
  milk
4 wild-caught cod fillets
  (or other firm, white
  fish), pin bones and skin
  removed, cut into large
  pieces
2 anchovies, finely
  chopped
2 cups snow pea pods,
  trimmed
1 tablespoon liquid
  coconut aminos
1 tablespoon wheat-free
  tamari or additional
  liquid coconut aminos
  for soy-free
5 makrut lime leaves,
  thinly sliced
4 cups cooked brown rice,
  for serving
Chopped fresh cilantro,
  for garnish

### STEPS

1.  To make the lime curry paste, using a mortar and pestle, pound the chives, ginger, lemongrass, honey, olive oil, curry powder, turmeric, and lime zest to a smooth paste.

2.  Melt the coconut oil in a wok or large skillet over medium heat. Add the curry paste and cook, stirring constantly, for 3 to 4 minutes, until fragrant.

3.  Stir in the coconut milk and bring to a simmer.

4.  Add the fish, anchovies, snow peas, coconut aminos, tamari or coconut aminos, and lime leaves. Stir and simmer for 3 minutes, or until the fish is just cooked through.

5.  Serve immediately over the brown rice, garnished with cilantro.

*Adapt It: For a Mild version with extra flavor, you can substitute 1 tablespoon garlic-infused olive oil for extra virgin olive oil.*

## Slow-Scrambled Eggs, Mushrooms & Greens Ⓜ ⑪
Serves 2

**INGREDIENTS**

2 tablespoons extra virgin olive oil, divided in half
8–10 shitake mushrooms, stems removed
Pinch sea salt and freshly ground black pepper
4 asparagus spears
4 large pasture-raised eggs
1 teaspoon grated lemon zest
½ teaspoon ground turmeric
Chopped fresh basil, for garnish

**STEPS**

1. Heat 1 tablespoon of the oil in a medium skillet over medium heat. Add the mushrooms and sprinkle with salt and pepper. Cook for 3 minutes, then add the asparagus and cook for about 6 minutes, until the mushrooms have softened and the asparagus is tender-crsip and brightened in color. Transfer the mushrooms and asparagus to a plate and tent with aluminum foil to keep warm.

2. Whisk the eggs in a bowl until nice and fluffy. Add the lemon zest and turmeric and blend thoroughly.

3. Heat the remaining 1 tablespoon oil in the same skillet over medium heat. Pour in the eggs, then turn the heat down to low. Add a pinch of salt and pepper.

4. With a flat-edged wooden spoon, stir gently and evenly, dragging the spoon across the entire bottom of the pan until cooked to your liking, 3 to 5 minutes.

5. Tumble the eggs out of the pan and serve with the mushrooms and asparagus, garnished with basil.

## Grass-Fed Lamb Lettuce Leaf Tacos Ⓜ
Makes 3 to 4 servings

### INGREDIENTS

1 tablespoon extra virgin olive oil
1 red onion, diced
2 garlic cloves, minced
1 pound organic ground lamb or beef
1 teaspoon smoked paprika, or to taste
Pinch dried chili flakes
1 tablespoon tomato paste
1 small bunch spinach, chopped
1 zucchini, grated
1 tomato, diced
2 scallions, chopped
Sea salt and freshly ground black pepper, to taste
6 large Boston lettuce leaves
1 avocado, peeled, pitted, and mashed or sliced lengthwise
½ cup plain, full-fat additive-free Greek yogurt (optional)
2 tablespoons nutritional yeast flakes (optional)

### STEPS

1. Heat the oil in a large skillet over medium heat. Add the onion and garlic and cook, stirring occasionally, for 5 minutes.

2. Add the ground lamb, paprika, and chili flakes and cook, using a wooden spoon to break up the meat, for 10 minutes.

3. Add the tomato paste, spinach, zucchini, tomato, and scallions and cook, stirring occasionally, for 15 minutes. Season with sea salt and pepper.

4. Place the lettuce leaves on a plate. Scoop up the meat and vegetable mixture and divide it between the leaves, taking care not to overfill them (so there is enough leaf to close up when eating).

5. Top each with a spoonful of mashed or sliced avocado and a teaspoon of Greek yogurt (if using), and garnish with a sprinkle of yeast flakes (if using).

## Sunday Braised Lamb on Butternut Squash Mash ⓜ

Serves 4 (with leftovers for lamb salad, page 198)

### INGREDIENTS

**Braised Lamb**

1 (4-pound) organic, grass-fed lamb shoulder or leg of lamb
4 garlic cloves, sliced
1 tablespoon basil leaves
Celtic sea salt and freshly ground pepper, to taste
1 tablespoon extra virgin olive oil
1 onion, cut into wedges
3 small carrots, halved lengthwise
1 red bell pepper, seeded and thinly sliced lengthwise
1 cup lamb bone broth (page 184 or store-bought)
1 tablespoon apple cider vinegar
¼ cup lemon juice, plus 2 lemon wedges
2 tablespoons dried oregano
Fresh flat-leaf parsley sprigs, for garnish

**Butternut Squash Mash**

½ butternut squash, halved and seeded
3 tablespoons extra virgin olive oil
2 garlic cloves, peeled
Celtic sea salt and freshly ground pepper, to taste
2 tablespoons chopped fresh flat-leaf parsley

### STEPS

1. First, start the lamb. Make four incisions into the lamb with a sharp knife, insert the garlic and basil into the incisions, and season generously with salt and pepper.

2. In a large ceramic Dutch oven, heat the oil over medium-high heat. Add the lamb and sear for 3 minutes on each side. Transfer the lamb to a plate.

3. Add the onion to the casserole dish and cook for 4 minutes.

4. Add the carrots, bell pepper, broth, vinegar, and lemon juice. Return the lamb to the casserole dish. Reduce the heat to very low, cover, and simmer for 1 hour.

5. Meanwhile, make the butternut squash. Preheat the oven to 350°F.

6. Put the squash, cut side up, in a baking dish. Pour the olive oil into the cavity and add the garlic cloves. Season with salt and pepper. Roast for about 1½ hours, until softened.

7. Once the lamb has cooked for 1 hour, turn it over, cover the dish again, and cook for another 1 hour. Add the lemon wedges and oregano and simmer for a final 30 minutes; the lamb should be tender and falling off the bone. Transfer the lamb to a cutting board and garnish with the parsley sprigs. Slice at the table.

8.  When the squash is done, use two forks to shred the flesh, making sure not to pierce the skin. Scoop the squash into a serving bowl. Garnish with chopped parsley and serve along with the lamb.

> **GutSMART Tips:**
>
> - To time your preparation so that both the lamb and mash are ready together, prepare the butternut squash as soon as you start cooking the lamb, then put it in the oven once you've turned the lamb and returned it to the heat for the second hour.
>
> - Celery root (aka celeriac) is a nice substitute for the butternut squash for a change of pace. It has a mild, celery-like flavor that sweetens with baking.

# SENSATIONAL SIDES

*Who doesn't love a flavorful side dish, like Turmeric Cauliflower (see color insert), as a complement to their meal? These sides are so good, you'll be going back for seconds. You can even serve the Good Gut Falafel Grazing Board with Dips (see color insert) as an hors d'oeuvre at your next dinner party.*

## Sweet Herb-Roasted Carrots S

Makes 2 servings

**INGREDIENTS**

6 thyme or lemon thyme sprigs
2 tablespoons extra virgin olive oil
1 tablespoon honey (optional; omit if fructose-intolerant)
1 tablespoon lemon juice
1 teaspoon fennel seeds
Sea salt and freshly ground black pepper, to taste
1 pound baby carrots, peeled and trimmed

**STEPS**

1. Preheat the oven to 400°F.

2. Combine the thyme, olive oil, honey (if using), lemon juice, fennel seeds, salt, and pepper in a small bowl and stir well.

3. Spread out the carrots in a large roasting pan, drizzle with the dressing, and toss to combine.

4. Roast for 25 to 30 minutes, until the carrots are cooked through.

## Crispy Sweet Potato Fries Ⓜ ✑

Makes 2 to 3 servings

**INGREDIENTS**

2 tablespoons avocado oil
1½ teaspoons almond meal
2 teaspoons fresh or dried rosemary
1 heaping teaspoon ground turmeric
½ teaspoon sweet paprika
1 teaspoon Celtic sea salt
Freshly cracked black pepper, to taste
1 large sweet potato, peeled and cut into ½-inch-thick fries
Homemade pesto (page 220), for serving (optional)

**STEPS**

1. Preheat the oven to 400°F.

2. Mix the avocado oil, almond meal, rosemary, turmeric, paprika, salt, and a good grind of pepper together in a large bowl. Add the sweet potato fries and stir until coated.

3. Spread out the fries on a rimmed baking sheet so they are not touching. Bake for 40 to 45 minutes, until crispy.

4. Serve warm, with pesto for dipping if desired.


## Broccoli & Peas with Hazelnuts, Lemon & Mint Ⓜ ✑

Makes 2 servings

**INGREDIENTS**

1 small head broccoli, roughly chopped
⅓ cup fresh or frozen peas
2 tablespoons extra virgin olive oil
Celtic sea salt
1 handful fresh mint leaves
1 tablespoon lemon juice
¼ cup hazelnuts, crushed, or toasted sprouted sunflower seeds

**STEPS**

1. Steam the broccoli and peas over boiling water for 5 minutes, until tender. Drain.

2. Heat the olive oil in a large skillet over medium heat. Add the broccoli and peas, sprinkle with a pinch of salt, and cook, stirring occasionally, for 1 to 2 minutes, or until cooked through.

3. Add the mint and lemon juice, sprinkle with the hazelnuts, and serve hot.

## 📷 Good Gut Falafel‡ Grazing Board with Dips Ⓜ 🔗 🕦

Makes 4 servings

### INGREDIENTS

#### Falafel

8 ounces dried chickpeas
1 teaspoon baking soda
2 cups mixed fresh cilantro, flat-leaf parsley, and mint leaves
6 scallions, white and pale green parts only, sliced
2 garlic cloves, minced
1 teaspoon ground cumin
½ teaspoon ground coriander
2 teaspoons sea salt, plus more for seasoning
2 to 3 cups refined avocado oil

#### Homemade Pesto

1 cup blanched almonds
3 large handfuls basil leaves, plus more for garnish
⅓ cup extra virgin olive oil, plus more for drizzling
1 teaspoon lemon zest
1 tablespoon lemon juice
2 tablespoons nutritional yeast flakes
Celtic sea salt

#### Green Bean Salsa

1 cup steamed green beans
1 red bell pepper, seeded and chopped
1 small handful mint leaves, plus more for garnish

½ teaspoon sweet paprika
1 tablespoon extra virgin olive oil, plus more for drizzling
Celtic sea salt and freshly cracked black pepper, to taste

#### Dippables

2 large pasture-raised eggs, soft-boiled for 4 minutes, peeled, and halved
2 carrots, peeled and cut into sticks
1 large cucumber, cut into sticks
Buckwheat Crackers (page 222)

### STEPS

1. Put the chickpeas in a large bowl. Cover with cold water and add the baking soda. Cover with a towel and let stand at room temperature overnight. The next day, drain, rinse, and carefully dry the chickpeas by putting them on a clean towel-lined baking sheet. Set aside to dry completely, about 1 hour.

2. Meanwhile, make the pesto. Put the almonds in a food processor and blend until fine. Add the basil and blend again. With the motor running, slowly drizzle in the olive oil until the desired consistency is reached. Add the lemon zest and juice, nutritional yeast, and a small pinch of salt. Transfer to a serving bowl.

---

‡ Recipe adapted from J. Kenji López-Alt. "Easy, Herb-Packed Falafel Recipe." Accessed March 24, 2022, from https://www.seriouseats.com/the-food-lab-vegan-experience -best-homemade-falafel-recipe.

3. Next, make the salsa. Steam the green beans over boiling water for 5 to 7 minutes, until tender. Drain. Clean out the food processor and add the beans, bell pepper, mint, paprika, and oil and process until finely chopped. Season with salt and pepper. Transfer to another serving bowl.

4. When ready to make the falafel, combine the chickpeas, herbs, scallions, garlic, cumin, coriander, and salt in a food processor. Pulse the mixture until it turns into a coarse meal, stopping the food processor to scrape down the sides as necessary. When squeezed into a ball, a handful of the mixture should almost be able to hold together. If not, process a little more.

5. Transfer to a bowl, cover, and place in the refrigerator for 15 minutes.

6. Scoop out a heaping tablespoon of the mixture into your hand (don't use too much or your falafel will fall apart). Gently shape each into a ball and place on a clean plate. Line a second plate with parchment paper.

7. Pour ¾ inch avocado oil into a deep cast-iron or nonstick skillet or Dutch oven. Heat over high heat until the oil reaches 375°F. Working in batches as necessary, carefully lower each chickpea ball into the oil with a slotted spoon, allowing a little space between them. Adjust the heat as necessary to maintain a temperature of between 350 and 375°F.

8. Allow the falafel to cook undisturbed until well browned on the bottom, then carefully flip the balls with a fork and cook until browned on the second side, about 4 minutes total.

9. Transfer the falafel to the parchment-lined plate. Sprinkle with salt immediately, while still hot. Repeat with the remaining chickpea balls.

10. Arrange the falafel and dippables on a large platter, with the dips alongside. Garnish the dips with chopped fresh herbs and a drizzle of olive oil.

**GutSMART Tip:** *Soaked then dried chickpeas—rather than canned—are essential to creating light and crispy falafel. Using dried chickpeas also eliminates the need for flour or other binders, making it more gut-friendly. And don't cook the dried chickpeas before making the falafel because you'll run into the same issues you find with canned—they just don't bind. The key to great falafel is to soak the dried chickpeas, let them air-dry, then grind them while they're still completely raw. They will cook in the next step, so you don't have to worry about getting the perfect result!*

# Baked Thyme Feta & Sardines with Buckwheat Crackers Ⓜ ⓪ⓘ

Makes 2 servings

## INGREDIENTS

### Buckwheat Crackers

4½ tablespoons buckwheat flour
½ cup ground flaxseed
1 tablespoon dried Italian herb seasoning
1 teaspoon grated lemon zest
½ teaspoon Celtic sea salt or pink Himalayan salt
2 medium pasture-raised eggs
1½ teaspoons extra virgin olive oil
1 tablespoon water (optional)

### Feta

1 (4-ounce) block feta cheese
¼ cup extra virgin olive oil
1 tablespoon lemon juice, plus lemon wedges for serving (optional)
1 teaspoon grated lemon zest
3 tablespoons fresh or dried thyme

### Sardines

1 (4-ounce) can sardines in olive oil
2 teaspoons apple cider vinegar
1 tablespoon lemon juice
Celtic sea salt and freshly ground black pepper, to taste

## STEPS

1. Preheat the oven to 350°F. Grease a rimmed baking sheet.

2. First, make the crackers. In a medium bowl, combine the buckwheat flour, flaxseed, Italian herbs, lemon zest, and salt.

3. In a small bowl, whisk together the eggs and olive oil.

4. Pour the egg mixture into the flour mixture and mix to form a dough. If it's too dry to roll out, mix in the water.

5. Roll out the dough on a sheet of parchment paper into a thin rectangle about 10 x 14 inches. Place the prepared baking sheet facedown over the dough, then invert the two together so the dough is on top. Peel off the parchment.

6. Using a sharp knife, cut the dough into 2-inch triangles or squares. (Alternatively, you can leave it whole and break into pieces once baked.)

7. Bake for 12 to 15 minutes, until crisp, turning the crackers over halfway through. Set aside the crackers to cool. Leave the oven on.

8. While the crackers are cooling, place the feta in a small baking dish. Pour the olive oil and lemon juice over the feta. Sprinkle with the lemon zest and thyme.

9. Bake for about 20 minutes, until the feta is hot and bubbling and slightly browned at the edges.

10. Put the sardines in a bowl. Add the vinegar, lemon juice, a pinch of salt, and pepper. Using a fork, gently mix to combine, lightly mashing the sardines if you like.

11. Serve the feta and sardines on the crackers, with lemon wedges if desired.

## Turmeric Cauliflower Ⓜ

Makes 4 servings

### INGREDIENTS

3 tablespoons extra virgin olive oil
2 tablespoons lemon juice, plus lemon wedges, for serving
2 garlic cloves, minced
2 tablespoons nutritional yeast flakes
1 teaspoon ground turmeric
1 teaspoon ground cumin
Sea salt and freshly ground black pepper, to taste
1 large head cauliflower, cut into florets
Chopped fresh cilantro, for garnish (optional)

### STEPS

1. Preheat the oven to 400°F. Line a rimmed baking sheet with parchment paper.

2. In a large bowl, whisk together the olive oil, lemon juice, garlic, nutritional yeast, turmeric, cumin, salt, and pepper. Add the cauliflower and mix until evenly coated.

3. Transfer the cauliflower to the prepared baking sheet.

4. Bake for 25 to 35 minutes, until tender, stirring twice for even cooking. Serve warm, with lemon wedges and fresh cilantro on top, if you like.

## Pistachio Portobello Mushrooms Ⓜ 🔗

Makes 4 servings

### INGREDIENTS

4 portobello mushrooms
or 8 button mushrooms,
stemmed
2 tablespoons wheat-free
tamari or liquid coconut
aminos for soy-free
3 tablespoons extra
virgin olive oil, divided
(2 tablespoons + 1
tablespoon)
1 tablespoon apple cider
vinegar
1 tablespoon lemon juice
2 garlic cloves, minced
⅓ cup chopped fresh
cilantro
¾ cup finely chopped
pistachios
Freshly cracked black
pepper, to taste

### STEPS

1. Put the mushrooms in a large bowl, cover with hot water, and let soak for 1 minute. Drain and pat dry with a paper towel.

2. In a small bowl, whisk together the tamari or coconut aminos, 2 tablespoons of the olive oil, the vinegar, lemon juice, garlic, and cilantro. Add the mushrooms and stir to ensure they are all coated. Cover and let marinate in the fridge for 1 hour.

3. Preheat the oven to 350°F.

4. In a small bowl, mix the pistachios, remaining 1 tablespoon olive oil, and pepper.

5. Place the mushrooms, stemmed side up, on a rimmed baking sheet. Spoon the pistachio mixture into each mushroom cap.

6. Bake for 20 minutes. Serve warm.

# FERMENTED DELIGHTS

*Fermented delights are a treat for a gut on its way to healing. They must be avoided if you're in the Severe category, but otherwise are a great adjunct to any gut-healing plan. Ferments improve the diversity of the gut microbiome and help reduce inflammation.*

## 📷 Cultured Carrot & Cabbage Ⓜ Ⓜ
Makes 4 pints

### INGREDIENTS

1 small red cabbage, shredded
1 medium carrot, peeled and shredded
2 teaspoons peeled and grated ginger
6 cups filtered water
1 tablespoon caraway seeds*
1 tablespoon Celtic sea salt
Freshly cracked black pepper

***Adapt It:** For a Moderate version, omit the caraway seeds.*

### STEPS

1. In a large bowl, combine the cabbage, carrot, and ginger. Divide the vegetables into 4 sterilized pint-size mason jars.

2. Pour the water into a pitcher and add the caraway seeds, salt, and a grind of pepper. Stir until the salt is dissolved.

3. Divide the water among the jars. Using a wooden spoon, push the vegetables down to ensure they're submerged and to remove any air pockets. There should be 1¼ inches space at the top of each jar to allow for expansion during fermentation. Put the lids on and seal tightly. Write the date on each jar.

4. Leave in a cool, dark, dry place for 3 to 5 days, until bubbles have started to form. Transfer to the fridge and enjoy for up to 1 month.

*GutSMART Tip: Double or triple the ingredients to prepare extra jars for the next two weeks.*

## 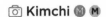 Kimchi Ⓜ Ⓜ

Makes about 4 cups

### INGREDIENTS

1 small green cabbage, shredded
1 turnip, peeled and grated
1 medium carrot, peeled and shredded
¾ cup grated zucchini
1 shallot, chopped fine
1 inch knob ginger, peeled and grated
1 garlic clove, crushed
1 heaping tablespoon chili flakes (optional)*
1 tablespoon caraway seeds (optional)*
1 tablespoon finely ground Celtic sea salt
Pinch freshly cracked black pepper

*Adapt It: For a non-spicy Moderate version, omit the chili flakes and caraway seeds.

### STEPS

1. In a large bowl, combine the cabbage, turnip, carrot, zucchini, shallot, ginger, garlic, chili flakes (if using), caraway seeds (if using), salt, and pepper. Using your hands, massage the seasonings into the vegetables until softened, about 4 minutes.

2. Set aside for 1 hour to allow the salt to draw the moisture out of the vegetables.

3. Transfer the vegetable mixture to a sterilized quart-size mason jar. Using a wooden spoon, push the mixture down firmly to remove any air pockets. There should be 1 inch space at the top to allow for expansion during fermentation. Put the lid on and seal tightly. Write the date on the jar.

4. Leave in a cool, dark, dry place for 3 to 5 days, until bubbles start to form. Transfer to the fridge and enjoy for up to 2 months.

*GutSMART Tip:* For easy-to-use fermentation compression lids with gas release that fit any wide-mouth mason jar, check out one of my favorite brands at **Krautsource.com**.

# Fermented Berries with Coconut or Greek Yogurt Ⓜ

Makes 1 pint

## INGREDIENTS

2½ cups mixed fresh
   berries
3 tablespoons filtered
   water
2 tablespoons maple
   syrup
1 teaspoon alcohol-free
   vanilla flavoring
½ teaspoon starter
   culture, or as instructed
   on package instructions
½ teaspoon Celtic sea salt
Coconut or Greek yogurt,
   for serving

## STEPS

1. Put the berries in a sterilized pint-size mason jar, pushing them down to fit.

2. In a small cup, mix together the water, maple syrup, vanilla, starter culture, and sea salt until the salt has dissolved.

3. Pour the liquid over the berries. Use a wooden spoon to push the berries down to ensure they're submerged and to remove any air pockets. There should be 1 inch space at the top of the jar to allow for expansion during fermentation.

4. Cover the jar with a square of cheesecloth, then screw the lid on tightly. Write the date on the jar.

5. Leave in a cool, dark, dry place for 1 to 2 days, until bubbles start to form. Transfer to the fridge and enjoy for up to 1 month.

6. To serve, scoop some Greek or coconut yogurt into a bowl and top with some fermented berries.

*GutSMART Tip:* Starter culture is sold online and at health food stores.

# DELECTABLE DESSERTS

*Although added sugar can be your gut's worst enemy, especially if you have underlying yeast overgrowth, everyone needs a little treat now and again. It's even better when it's a guilt-free dessert that makes you feel like you're cheating without cheating. Your mouth will be watering when you see the delicious Nutty Apple Crumble (see color insert). And the refreshing dairy-free Lemon & Berry Gelato makes for a nice treat on a hot summer afternoon.*

## Kiwi & Pineapple Rice Pudding ⓢ

Makes 2 servings

### INGREDIENTS

1 (13.5-ounce) can additive-free coconut milk
¼ cup white rice
1 tablespoon coconut sugar
1 teaspoon alcohol-free vanilla flavoring
Pinch sea salt
Pinch ground cinnamon
1 star anise pod
1 kiwifruit, peeled and sliced
½ cup pineapple chunks

### STEPS

1.  In a medium saucepan, bring the coconut milk to a gentle boil over medium heat.

2.  Reduce the heat to low and stir in the rice. Add the coconut sugar, vanilla, sea salt, cinnamon, and star anise and cook for about 25 minutes, until the rice is tender and creamy.

3.  Spoon into bowls and top with kiwi slices and pineapple chunks.

## Berry-Lime Pudding Ⓜ ✏

Makes 2 servings

### INGREDIENTS

2 cups frozen raspberries
  and blueberries
20 macadamia nuts,
  soaked in water for 1
  hour and drained
20 hazelnuts, soaked in
  water for 1 hour and
  drained
½ cup additive-free
  coconut milk
Grated zest and juice of
  1 lime
½ teaspoon alcohol-free
  vanilla flavoring
½ teaspoon allulose or
  ¼ teaspoon stevia
Small pinch Celtic sea salt

### STEPS

Puree all the ingredients in a food processor until smooth and creamy. Serve immediately.

## Lemon & Berry Gelato Ⓜ

Makes 2 servings

### INGREDIENTS

1 cup frozen blueberries
½ medium avocado,
  pitted and peeled
½ cup ice cubes
¼ cup additive-free
  coconut milk
Juice of ½ lemon
½ teaspoon alcohol-free
  vanilla flavoring
Fresh mint leaves, for
  garnish

### STEPS

Puree the blueberries, avocado, ice cubes, coconut milk, lemon, and vanilla in a blender until smooth and creamy. Garnish with mint leaves and serve immediately.

## 📷 Nutty Apple Crumble Ⓜ 🔗 🗍

Makes 6 servings

### INGREDIENTS

- 4–5 Granny Smith apples, cored and sliced into thin half-moons
- 2 tablespoons coconut sugar
- 1 teaspoon ground nutmeg
- 1 teaspoon ground cinnamon
- 1 teaspoon lemon juice
- ½ cup dry-roasted almonds
- 3½ ounces hazelnuts
- 3½ ounces pistachios
- 4 tablespoons unsalted grass-fed butter, cut into cubes
- Pinch Celtic sea salt
- 1 tablespoon honey
- Plain Greek or coconut yogurt, for serving

### STEPS

1. Preheat the oven to 350°F. Grease an 8-inch square baking dish.

2. In a bowl, toss the apples with the coconut sugar, nutmeg, cinnamon, and lemon juice until evenly coated.

3. Layer the apple slices in the prepared baking dish.

4. In a food processor, pulse the almonds, hazelnuts, and pistachios until roughly chopped, then remove one-quarter of the nut mixture and set aside.

5. Add the butter and salt to the nuts remaining in the food processor. Pulse until crumbly.

6. Sprinkle the butter-nut mixture over the apples, top with the reserved nuts, and drizzle with the honey.

7. Bake for 25 minutes, or until crispy on top. Add a dollop of yogurt on top and serve warm.

# Metric Conversion Table

## Abbreviation key

tsp = teaspoon

tbsp = tablespoon

dsp = dessert spoon

| US Standard | UK |
|---|---|
| ¼ tsp | ¼ tsp (scant) |
| ½ tsp | ½ tsp (scant) |
| ¾ tsp | ½ tsp (rounded) |
| 1 tsp | ¾ tsp (slightly rounded) |
| 1 tbsp | 2½ tsp |
| ¼ cup | ¼ cup minus 1 dsp |
| ⅓ cup | ¼ cup plus 1 tsp |
| ½ cup | ⅓ cup plus 2 dsp |
| ⅔ cup | ½ cup plus 1 tbsp |
| ¾ cup | ½ cup plus 2 tbsp |
| 1 cup | ¾ cup and 2 dsp |

# PART IV

........................................

# TURBOCHARGING YOUR RESULTS

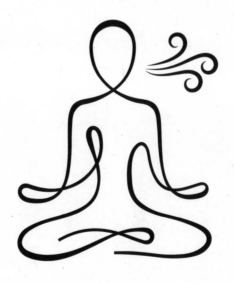

# Chapter 10

# THE VAGUS NERVE: YOUR GUT IS CALLING

> *"The vagus nerve is like a telephone wire between the gut and the brain, allowing them to communicate with each other."*
>
> —Dr. Vincent Pedre

**By this point, you've ingested a lot of information. You have learned** about the gut, microbiome, and digestion, received your GutSMART Quiz results, and familiarized yourself with your individualized meal plan and the recipes. Congratulations—you are doing the work! All the knowledge you have gained thus far will set you on a path towards healing your gut and, in the process, restoring your body to its ideal state of health. And now you've reached Part IV of this book, which I named "Turbocharging Your Results" for one important reason: I didn't want you to miss it!

You see, most people never get this far into a book. They usually stop reading after the first couple of chapters. That's why I wanted to lure you here with a promise: If you read and implement the practices in the next few chapters, you're going to *turbocharge your results*! Who would want to miss out on that opportunity?! In the next three chapters, I'll walk you through methods and practices you can integrate into your life to both accelerate and prolong your gut-healing results. These are like extra credit, but in my experience and that of my clients, they make a *huge* difference.

The first way to turbocharge your results is by harnessing the power of your **vagus nerve**. In this chapter, I'll bring you up to speed on the vagus nerve and what it does, and give you practical advice on how you can stimulate yours to improve both your gut health and general well-being.

# VAGUS 101

Let's take it from the top: What is the vagus nerve? The vagus nerve is the longest nerve in the body, and even though we don't hear about it very often, it's an essential player in the gut-brain connection.

The vagus nerve runs from the base of the brain, down the neck, and along the spine, and interacts with most major organs, including the gut. It's one of the main components of the parasympathetic nervous system (PNS), otherwise known as the "rest and digest" system.

## Sympathetic vs. Parasympathetic Nervous Systems

A little science class refresher: The **autonomic nervous system** (ANS) is the part of the nervous system that controls things like your heart rate and the contraction of your blood vessels, seemingly independent of conscious thought. It is divided into two parts: the sympathetic nervous system and the parasympathetic nervous system. The **sympathetic nervous system** regulates our "fight or flight" response—its job is to increase blood circulation throughout the body to support movement.[1] The **parasympathetic nervous system**, on the other hand, supports health, growth, and restoration. It helps return your body to homeostasis after stressful situations—it brings your heart rate down and returns your body to a calm and content state (which is ideal for digestion!).

In his book *The Pocket Guide to Polyvagal Theory*, psychiatrist and neuroscientist Stephen W. Porges explains that the vagus nerve has motor pathways that go from the brain to the organs, as well as sensory pathways running from the organs to the brain. **Polyvagal theory**, the central concept of his book, asserts that our organs are not independent structures "unconnected and uninformed by brain processes."[2] Instead, our visceral organs have a direct impact on brain processes, just as our brain processes have an impact on our visceral organs. It's essentially a two-way street.

Put simply, the vagus nerve connects the brain to the rest of the body. And the gut, which contains the second biggest nervous system in the body (aka the **enteric nervous system**, or ENS), is at the center of that connection. The gut microbiota communicate with the brain via their interactions with the ENS and most importantly, the vagus nerve.[3] I know that may sound confusing, so here's a diagram:

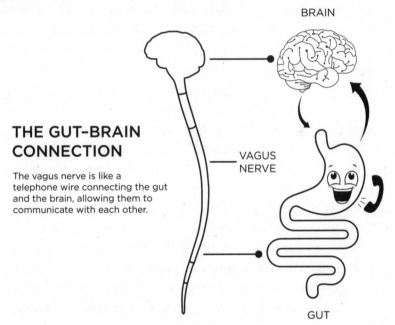

BRAIN

**THE GUT–BRAIN CONNECTION**

The vagus nerve is like a telephone wire connecting the gut and the brain, allowing them to communicate with each other.

VAGUS NERVE

GUT

As the central component of the parasympathetic nervous system, the vagus nerve influences a wide range of bodily functions, including:[4]

- Gut permeability (how tight or "leaky" your gut barrier is)
- Gut motility (the rhythmic contractions of your digestive system)
- Digestion (enzyme secretion and stomach acid levels)
- Immunity
- Stress response
- Mood and mental health
- Heart rate and *heart rate variability*

(**Heart rate variability** [**HRV** for short] is a measure of the variation in time between your heartbeats. Simply put, your heart doesn't beat in a steady rhythm. It changes, beat to beat. Why is the variation in the intervals between those beats so important? HRV is controlled by the autonomic nervous system, which also regulates your heart rate, blood pressure, digestion, and even breathing rate. HRV is directly influenced by sympathetic and parasympathetic firing of the ANS. In other words, HRV is a measure of how balanced your autonomic nervous system is.[5])

As you can see, the vagus nerve plays a varied and significant role in the body, and because of that, it's extremely important. So important, in fact, that it baffles me how few people know about it! Unless you're very clued in to the world of gut health, or you're a physician yourself, this may be the first time you're hearing about the vagus nerve. *Why is this?* Well, while there is a growing body of research underscoring all of the functions of the vagus nerve, we're still figuring out how it works exactly. Don't get me wrong, we know *a lot*, but there's much more to learn. As for what we do know, for whatever reason, this knowledge wasn't trickling down from medical and research circles to the general population *up until now*. No matter—by the end of this chapter, you'll know plenty about the vagus nerve.

## Think of the vagus nerve as a telephone wire that allows your brain and gut to communicate with each other.

It's through the vagus nerve that the microbes in your gut communicate with your brain and central nervous system. We tend to think of the brain as the control center—the head honcho that doles out orders to the rest of the body. As you've learned, though, *it all starts in the gut*. To use the telephone metaphor: If the gut and the brain are on the phone with each other (think pre–cell phone age, when telephones needed wires to work), the gut is the one doing most of the talking. That's because most of the nerves that make up the vagus fire upstream to the brain, not downstream from the brain to the gut. In fact, 80 to 90 percent of the fibers in the vagus nerve point up towards the brain.[6] So the majority of the time, the gut is relaying information to the brain—meaning your gut plays a key role in your thoughts.

Research has shown that the better your vagus nerve is functioning, the more capable you are of regulating your stress response. Pretty wild, isn't it? The nerve endings of the vagus nerve in the gut have receptors known as **5-HT receptors** (5-HT is 5-hydroxytryptophan), whose job it is to sense **serotonin** (your "happiness molecule") secreted by gut bacteria and, in response, send a signal to the brain, via the vagus nerve, to release **GABA** (a natural brain relaxant) in brain regions that control nerve activation. (We're taught that serotonin is a brain chemical that's only produced by the brain when in reality, gut bacteria manufacture about 95 percent of the body's supply of serotonin.) When your brain nerve cells are overactivated, you may experience symptoms like anxiety or attention deficit hyperactivity disorder.

## The main job of the vagus nerve is to survey and send information about our organs back to our brain. If something is off in the gut, the vagus nerve carries that information back to the brain.

What this means is that the gut can have a direct impact on your mental state. The information the brain receives from the gut and gut microbiome via the vagus nerve can end up influencing your mood, anxiety levels, and even mental health. Yes, I said it: Depression could be tied to the state of your gut and gut microbiome. Happiness truly does start in the gut!

# HOW THE VAGUS NERVE AFFECTS GUT HEALTH

Okay, so we've discussed how the vagus nerve affects the body and how it serves as a way for the gut and brain to chitchat, as well as how your gut health affects your brain through it. But how does the vagus nerve actually impact your gut health?

Great question! When your vagus nerve is functioning properly (something we call good **vagal tone**—think dial tone on the now-antique, wired telephone), it helps maintain the integrity (or normal permeability) of your gut lining. Research has found that vagal nerve stimulation decreases intestinal permeability by increasing the expression of tight junction proteins along the cell membrane of intestinal cells.[7] In other words, it ensures that your gut interface is tightly sealed—that only dietary nutrients get into the rest of the body, while inflammatory substances and gut bugs are kept out. If you think back to the coffee filter analogy from chapter 1, good vagal tone is one of several important factors that help your gut keep the "coffee grounds" (bad gut bugs and *endotoxins*, discussed in chapter 2) out of your cup of coffee.

Issues arise, however, when your vagus nerve becomes dysfunctional as a result of stressful situations or traumatic head injury/concussion. When your vagus malfunctions, it can cause the gut to become more permeable. The gut barrier opens up, and endotoxins, bacteria, and other inflammation-provoking substances flood into the bloodstream, increasing your risk for the chronic degenerative diseases that are plaguing modern society. (For a refresher on leaky gut, flip back to page 22.)

As you have learned already, the gut affects every system in our bodies, and problems in the gut, like leaky gut syndrome, often lead to unwanted gut-related symptoms in other parts of the body, including serious health issues like auto-immune disease. Therefore, your digestion, immune system, mental health, and overall longevity—all the gut-health interrelationships we described in chapters 2 and 3—can be further compromised if the vagus nerve isn't functioning as intended. This underperformance, or **low vagal tone**, is an added factor that can aggravate all of the other underlying factors affecting the gut that we discussed earlier in this book.

# SIGNS YOUR VAGUS NERVE IS UNDERPERFORMING

Generally speaking, we could all benefit from *more vagal tone*. Most of us experience stress at unhealthy levels because our society praises productivity, requires constant engagement, and undervalues rest and recovery. We're taught to be efficient and maximize our output, and as a result, self-care falls by the wayside. Nowhere is this more apparent than in the data we have around mental health.

In 2017, an estimated 284 million people worldwide were diagnosed with an anxiety disorder, a number that has continued to grow.[8] And that's just anxiety! It was also estimated that a total of *792 million people* were struggling with a mental health disorder in 2017.[9] And those numbers inevitably increased exponentially during the global pandemic. In other words, our mental health demands our attention, and activating the vagus nerve can not only help mitigate stress but also alleviate anxiety and even "treatment-resistant" depression.

There are a few proven ways to increase vagus nerve activity. Under certain circumstances, like treatment-resistant depression, the use of medical vagus nerve stimulating devices has been shown to help. Yes, it's possible to stimulate the vagus nerve with electrical current. It's something often done in a doctor's office, but there are FDA-approved devices available for home use. One device, in particular, the *gammaCore*, is a noninvasive vagal nerve stimulation device that can be purchased over the counter and used without a doctor's supervision, and it has been approved by the FDA for treating migraines.[10] Another such handheld device is known as *NES miHealth*, and in one outcome study, 93 percent of participants using it reported a positive impact on chronic and acute pain, including stomach pain, and lower mental stress.[11] But most people will be able to stimulate their vagus nerve just fine by adding behavior-based activities to their daily routine, no electrical stimulation device needed. (I'll get into those in just a moment.)

In case you're curious what an underactive vagus nerve looks like—again, we call this **low vagal tone**—the following box shows some of the possible signs and symptoms. Many of these we know about because vagus nerve stimulation has been used successfully in the treatment of these conditions.

## Signs You May Be Suffering from Low Vagal Tone

Have you ever felt so anxious you had a "pit" in your stomach? Are you the type that loses your appetite when you're stressed? Does food not "sit well" when you're nervous, leaving you nauseated or feeling like it sits in your stomach for hours? These are all signs that your vagus nerve has been affected by stress. Low vagal tone leads to low stomach acid production, which makes it much more difficult to digest food properly—especially high-protein meals. As a result, the food will sit in your stomach for hours like a brick. Here are some other signs your vagus nerve may *not* be functioning properly:

- Increased response to stress (you get stressed easily, and you react intensely)
- Slow emotional and physiological recovery after stressors[12] (you have trouble regrounding yourself after a stressful situation)
- Poor emotional regulation (your emotions feel out of your control)[13]
- General anxiety[14]
- High levels of aggression[15]
- Depression[16]
- Fatigue[17]
- Headaches[18] and migraines[19]
- Abdominal pain[20]
- Heartburn/acid reflux[21]
- Constipation[22]
- Unexpected weight gain[23]
- Obesity[24]

It's also possible for your vagus nerve to be damaged, which often leads to **gastroparesis**—a condition that affects the smooth muscle of the stomach, both slowing down the emptying of your stomach and inhibiting proper digestion.[25]

While only an estimated 5 million people in the US have been formally diagnosed with gastroparesis,[26] symptoms of gastroparesis occur in about 1 in 4 adults in the US.[27] Damage to the vagus nerve is commonly caused by inflammatory diseases or surgery to the stomach or small intestine. Factors that can increase your risk of gastroparesis include:[28]

- Diabetes
- Abdominal or esophageal surgery
- Infection, usually from a virus
- Certain medications that slow the rate of stomach emptying, like narcotic pain meds
- Scleroderma (an autoimmune connective tissue disease)
- Nervous system diseases like Parkinson's disease and multiple sclerosis
- Hypothyroidism (underactive thyroid)

The take-home here? If your vagus is off, you're going to feel off. Digestion is going to run slow. And you may suffer from other health consequences, like depression, migraines, and/or constipation. So, it's important to consider the things you can do to increase vagal tone as part of any gut-healing protocol.

## WHAT YOU CAN DO TO STIMULATE THE VAGUS NERVE

So much of what your body does happens behind the scenes and without your conscious input. Think about when you have a common cold or a stomach bug—your body reacts without you having to lift a finger, and while sometimes it needs outside help (say, in the form of antibiotics), the body does a great deal on its own. When it comes to gut health, though, there's only so much the body can do, especially if it's also having to fix ongoing harm. For example, if you constantly eat a heavily processed, high-calorie, low-nutrient diet, your body will be continually working to counteract the new damage being inflicted on it. It won't have time to focus on getting back to homeostasis.

One big way you can lend your body a hand (beyond avoiding things that cause additional damage!) is to optimize how your vagus nerve functions. Fortunately, there are a multitude of ways to stimulate your vagus nerve naturally to improve your vagal tone and boost your gut-healing efforts tenfold!

## 7 Ways to Activate Your Vagus Nerve

1. **Find ways to de-stress.**

   Being chronically stressed means your autonomic nervous system is out of balance. Your sympathetic nervous system is constantly activated, so your body is always in fight-or-flight mode, overpowering your parasympathetic nervous system; therefore, your body is in a constant state of unrest. Have you ever heard the phrase "tired but wired"? If you find that you often have trouble winding down or relaxing, even when you're exhausted, chances are you're dealing with chronic stress.

   The vagus nerve is very sensitive, and chronic stress can cause it to malfunction, leaving you with a leaky gut and, by proxy, a host of other health problems. What's the solution? Find a way to de-stress! Different methods work for different people, but here are a few of my go-to stress hacks. Each of these takes only ten minutes, so I encourage you to experiment and try a bunch of them so you can see which work best for you.

---

### Ten-Minute Stress Hacks

- **Meditate.** More on this later! Chapter 12 is all about meditating, and I've brought in the best teachers out there to guide you.

- **Go for a mindful walk outside (that means drop the smartphone on your way out).** Or walk inside if outside isn't doable. Just get your body moving! Take care to be present with the moment to get the full effects (the breathwork in chapter 11 will help with this).

- **Stretch your full body.** Start with your shoulders, upper back, lower back, and hips—we hold a lot of tension in these areas.

---

- **Dance it out.** Dancing is an underrated movement exercise that has been shown to help us cope with depression, process stress, and move through grief.[29] Put on your favorite song, and let the music move your body.

- **Call or text a loved one.** Sometimes all we need is a little connection to make us feel relaxed and safe. Call a family member or friend who you know can give you reassurance and a sense of security.

- **Go for a bike ride.** Prolonged exercise gets your body to release those feel-good chemicals known as **endorphins**, which not only improve your mood but also lower your stress levels.[30] If you can ride your bike outside in nature, all the better!

- **Get ten minutes of sunlight.** Have you noticed the pattern? I'm telling you to get outside! Numerous studies have concluded that exposure to natural environments can reduce stress levels.[31] Even ten minutes of sunlight can make a difference.

- **Take a warm Epsom salt bath or go sweat in a sauna.** Taking a warm bath in Epsom salts has been shown to increase feelings of relaxation and relief.[32] (This is why hot springs offer a double whammy of benefits for your health—you get both a hot bath and exposure to nature.) The same goes for spending time in a sauna—it can produce feelings of tranquility and improve your mental well-being.[33]

2.  **Learn deep diaphragmatic breathing.**
    Breathing—specifically, *diaphragmatic or deep breathing*—is one of the most powerful tools you have for stimulating your vagus nerve. This type of breathing is often employed in meditation practices, and it's been shown to not only reduce stress levels and lower anxiety, but also

improve gastrointestinal function by way of the vagus nerve.[34] The great thing is, it's totally free, and you can take it with you wherever you go.

However, diaphragmatic breathing doesn't come naturally to most of us, so it can take a little practice. When you inhale, your belly should expand first, and when you exhale, it should retract back toward you. It looks like this: Breathe in, belly out. Breathe out, belly in.

In the next chapter, "Breathing Your Way to Gut Bliss," you'll find breathwork exercises from my favorite instructors. Mastering deep, diaphragmatic breathing will prepare you for the breathwork exercises coming up.

## A Deep-Diaphragmatic Breathing Primer

This is the way I teach my patients deep, diaphragmatic breathing:

1. Lie on your back on a well-supported surface, such as the floor or a bed, with knees bent and feet flat.

2. Put one hand on your belly and the other hand on your chest.

3. Take a deep breath in and let it out, becoming aware of how the breath moves in and out of your lungs, as well as how your hands move during the breath. (Does one hand move before the other? Which one?)

4. Relax your body and get ready to practice deep, diaphragmatic breathing.

5. Start by exhaling completely.

6. Then, breathe into the hand on your belly, expanding your belly as much as possible while breathing in.

7. As the bottom of your lungs fill and your belly expansion slows down, start filling your upper lungs with air as well,

feeling the hand on your chest move up and your back move toward the floor or bed.

8. Now reverse the order as you exhale, first breathing out from your chest, feeling the hand over your chest drop, then exhaling more deeply by contracting your abdominal muscles, feeling the hand on your belly drop as your belly button moves toward your back, squeezing all the air out of your lungs.

9. Repeat by following steps 6, 7, and 8 again.

10. Set a timer and do this for ten minutes. Let me know how you feel by visiting **GutSMARTProtocol.com** or send me a DM on Instagram **@drpedre**.

3. **Practice yoga.**

   Practices that incorporate gentle exercise and stretching have been shown to improve **peristalsis**—the rhythmic contractions of the intestinal smooth muscle that push the intestines' contents forward—by activating the vagus nerve. Among these, yoga is one of the best for stress and anxiety relief to improve gut function.[35] It also utilizes deep breathing! A true win-win. You can check out yoga poses for gut health in my first book, *Happy Gut*.

4. **Eat a diet rich in fermented foods.**

   Since their discovery thousands of years ago, we have known that fermented foods are an essential part of healthy living, but what many people don't know is that microorganisms in the gut (like those found in probiotic supplements and fermented foods) can stimulate the vagus nerve.[36] Strong evidence from animal studies has shown that one of the ways gut microorganisms have a direct influence on the brain and behavior is by activating the vagus nerve. (For more on how to incorporate fermented foods into your diet and to find out which ones are right for you, see chapter 7.)

5. **Sing your favorite song.**

   I know this one may seem random, but singing can boost your vagal tone! Listening to music alone has the ability to de-stress us, and when you add singing to the mix, it's a powerful stress-busting duo.[37] Studies have demonstrated that singing can decrease cortisol levels, but that's not all.[38] As Stephen W. Porges notes, singing can calm the whole body via the vagus nerve. The vagus nerve runs close to your vocal cords and the muscles at the back of your throat, which means the vibrations created by engaging them while singing will stimulate your vagus nerve.

   Singing also involves deep breathing. When you sing, you need to expand your ribcage and prolong the duration of your exhalation. During the exhalation phase of breathing, the tone of the vagal nerve fibers that signal from the brain to the periphery of the body (and especially the pathways to the heart) increase. (This explains how playing a wind instrument can contribute to a calmer physiological state, too!)[39]

   So next time you're feeling stress or anxiety building up in you, activate your vagus nerve by putting on a song you love and belting it out!

6. **Gargle water.**

   That's right, gargling can activate your vagus nerve. It almost sounds too good to be true because it's so simple. Similar to singing, gargling vibrates your vocal cords and the muscles at the back of your throat, stimulating the vagus nerve.[40] I recommend doing this exercise in the morning and in the evening when you're brushing your teeth—you'll be more likely to remember to do it because you'll be adding it to an already existing, consistent routine.

7. **Take a cold shower.**

   I know you're probably thinking, *Wait, didn't you just tell me to take a warm bath?* Yes, I did, but oddly enough, cold showering can activate the parasympathetic nervous system, too, which the vagus nerve is a part of![41] You don't have to take an exclusively cold shower (because really, who wants to do that?), but ending your shower with ninety seconds to two minutes of cold water can stimulate your vagus nerve by activating cold receptors in the face and neck and allowing your body to come out of fight-or-flight mode.[42]

## Takeaways

Woo-hoo! You now have even *more* tools in your gut-healing toolkit than you did before. In the next two chapters, you'll learn all about breathwork and meditation, so once you're done reading this chapter summary, take a step back, breathe, and keep going!

1.  The vagus nerve is at the heart of the gut-brain connection. It plays a critical role in the parasympathetic nervous system and influences a number of bodily functions, like digestion, gut permeability, stress response, mental health, and immunity.

2.  The vagus nerve is like a telephone wire—it allows your brain and gut to communicate with each other.

3.  Loss of vagal tone can cause issues in your gut, especially leaky gut syndrome.

4.  If you experience chronic or high levels of stress, anxiety, depression, aggression, or fatigue, you may have an underactive vagus nerve (that is, *low vagal tone*). Headaches, migraines, constipation, and acid reflux are also signs that your vagus nerve could benefit from stimulation using the techniques described in this chapter.

5.  There are hacks you can use to stimulate your vagus nerve naturally.

6.  Lowering your stress levels is crucial for good vagal tone and gut health. Activities like dancing, yoga, taking a nature walk, and deep breathing can help improve your vagal tone.

7.  Additionally, hot baths or cold showers, diets high in fermented foods and probiotics, singing, and gargling are powerful ways to activate your vagus nerve.

## Chapter 11

# BREATHING YOUR WAY TO GUT BLISS

> *"Where we send the breath is where we send function."*
>
> —Sachin Patel

**In the last chapter, I explained the important role the vagus nerve** plays in gut health, and together we laid down the cornerstone for the rest of Part IV —deep, diaphragmatic breathing. This chapter and the next will take you deeper into two essential tools—breathwork and meditation—that can give your gut a health boost by lowering your stress levels and getting you out of the fight-or-flight response cycle you've been living in. Let's start with breathwork.

Breathwork has been around for centuries, but only in the last decade has it started trickling down to the mainstream. In this chapter, I'll give you a crash course on breathwork, including what it is, how it helps the gut, and the research behind it. And best of all, I'll provide three different breathwork exercises specifically designed to improve your gut health, contributed by some of the best breathwork experts and coaches I've met throughout my career.

Each exercise comes with step-by-step instructions and is designed to let you practice it at home, on the go, or wherever you are. I've chosen these particular breathwork experts—Emily Fletcher, Jesse Gros, Lee Holden, and Sachin Patel—because they are at the forefront of their fields, share my passion for integrative wellness, and have dedicated their lives to helping people feel better through mindfulness practices. This chapter is packed with useful information and expertise . . . so let's get to it.

# WHAT IS BREATHWORK?

**Breathwork** is a term that refers to any kind of breathing technique or exercise. Every person you speak to will define breathwork differently, but one of my favorite explanations comes from Deepak Chopra:

> *Breathwork encompasses a broad range of whole-being therapeutic practices and exercises used to relieve mental, physical, and/or emotional tension. In the ancient yogic teachings, the practice of directing the breath is called Pranayama, and it teaches you to breathe consciously, with awareness, and with intent. Breathwork, though, is more than an exercise of breathing correctly or with intent. Breathing techniques are tools for major transformation and healing.*[1]

Most breathwork involves a form of breathing called *diaphragmatic breathing* (discussed in chapter 10). You may have heard this referred to as "belly breathing," "deep breathing," or "abdominal breathing." Let me share a little science to help you understand it better. You are probably already familiar with your diaphragm—the large, dome-shaped muscle below your lungs that contracts and expands as you breathe, helping you inhale and exhale. **Diaphragmatic breathing** is exactly what it sounds like: breathing with your diaphragm. When we're born, we instinctively breathe using our diaphragms, but as time goes on, that changes.

*Wait, I'm breathing the wrong way right now? What's the difference between diaphragmatic breathing and how I normally breathe?* Great questions! Unless you are actively practicing diaphragmatic breathing daily (because you're a yogi or a meditation teacher), it's likely that you are instead **chest breathing**: taking breaths using your chest and small accessory rib muscles. In other words, you're taking smaller, shorter, shallower breaths than you would if you were using diaphragmatic breathing. Chest breaths are unsatisfying because they don't allow for a complete oxygen exchange (inhaling oxygen and exhaling carbon dioxide). People tend to chest breathe when they're stressed, rushing, or busy.[2] But the other reason people become chest breathers is due to societal pressures to maintain the illusion of a thin waist—diaphragmatic breathing moves your stomach out while you're inhaling in a way chest breathing does not.

Unfortunately, sucking in the belly and chest breathing isn't great for your body. Using your neck, shoulders, and chest to breathe is not only inefficient, but also, in some ways, dangerous. Breathing this way often leads to headaches, injuries, and poor posture.[3] (I know! The breath is that powerful.)

When it comes to practicing breathwork, there are numerous methods, exercises, and techniques you can choose from, many of which also involve meditation (which you'll read more about in the next chapter). The goal, as Chopra notes, is to improve overall well-being, which includes our mental, physical, and spiritual selves. Many people like to practice breathwork with a coach or teacher, while others prefer the convenience and comfort of doing breathwork alone at home. Regardless of where or how you practice, the benefits of breathwork, particularly for your gut and digestion, are impressive and well researched.

## LIGHT YOUR DIGESTIVE FIRE
## WITH BREATHWORK

I sat down with my friend Lee Holden, internationally renowned expert and instructor in Qigong, a Chinese system of coordinated breath and movement exercises designed to optimize energy, health, and well-being, to ask him about the Chinese medicine perspective on the breath and digestion. Here's what he had to say:

> From a Chinese medicine perspective, gut health is compared to a fire. Your digestion, often referred to as metabolic fire, transforms food into energy. Think of your belly as the fire and the food you eat as the log you will put on that fire. If, for example, you have a weak fire and a wet log, the wood isn't going to transform into heat very easily. The wet log is akin to poor choices in food. Eating fast-food burgers and ice cream every day is like putting a wet log on that fire. Stress, antibiotics, and lack of exercise can cause a weak fire in your digestion. So can

*poor eating habits over time. This combination causes a lot of health issues in your whole system.*

*What does a fire need to thrive? Oxygen. If a fire gets weak, what do you do? You blow on it. You've done that at a bonfire, right? Fire starts to smolder, gets weak, you blow some $O_2$ on it, and the fire erupts from the logs. Well, your digestion works in much the same way.*

*Food would be useless without oxygen. I'm not talking about a metaphorical or Eastern medicine perspective. Without oxygen, your food would be inert, not usable to the cells in your body. Oxygen is essential for converting food energy into fuel for your body.*

This is one of many reasons breathwork is essential for a healthy digestive system. Not only that, but the *way* you breathe directly communicates to your nervous system which branch to activate. Shallow, quick chest breathing signals the body to trigger the sympathetic "fight or flight" branch. Slow, deep, relaxed breathing stimulates the parasympathetic "rest and digest" branch.

When you're under stress, shallow breathing is an evolutionary instinct that shunts blood flow away from your gut and to your muscles, so you're ready to move quickly under threat. Think of it this way: If you're being chased by a Rottweiler, digesting food isn't your body's highest priority; instead, all your energy is diverted to surviving. Digestion is put on pause until you are safe.

Lee further explained: "Your body doesn't know the difference between sitting in traffic, having a stressful meeting, financial pressure, or being attacked by a saber-toothed tiger. Even though your life isn't in danger with these day-to-day occurrences, your nervous system still allocates all of its resources to fight-or-flight. This leaves very little energy to devote to rest-and-digest."

What this means is that when you're experiencing chronic stress, your body interprets it the same way it would a threat to your life. Your breath becomes a mirror of how you are feeling internally. But while the breath follows what the brain feels, the reverse can *also* happen—the brain follows what the breath does.

"Think about how someone breathes when they are angry," Lee pointed out. "Strong exhales, shallow inhales. When someone is sad or crying: lots of exhaling and short gasping inhales. Breath reflects emotion. If we breathe slowly and deeply, we send a message to our nervous system that we are safe—a message to relax, be at peace, rest, and digest."

# HOW BREATHWORK CALMS THE GUT

In the interest of getting you to the breathwork exercises ASAP, I'll give you just a short spiel on how gut health and breathwork are connected. The research on breathwork and the gut is, to most people's surprise, extensive. In chapter 1, we covered how the gut is connected to every system in the body—like the brain, skin, and metabolism—and how it has a symbiotic relationship with many of them. We saw how this holds true for your respiratory system as well.[4] And in chapter 10 we saw how the gut is also affected by our breath, namely because the breath can take us out of fight-or-flight and activate the vagus nerve, helping us get into rest-and-digest mode. That means that breathwork can improve digestion when done both *before eating* and *after eating* (two of the exercises below will show you how).

Breathwork has numerous benefits for both the mind and body. People utilize breathwork daily to address issues from anxiety and anger to depression, grief, and post-traumatic stress disorder (PTSD), and even chronic pain.[5] Diaphragmatic breathing also works wonders for lowering your heart rate and blood pressure, as well as oxidative stress (think inflam-aging!).[6] As you learned in chapter 1, the gut is extremely sensitive to stress. It's common to experience physical symptoms like an upset stomach, abdominal pain, diarrhea, constipation, bloating, and IBS when you're stressed or anxious, so it makes sense that breathing in a way that lowers your stress levels is going to have a positive impact on gut health.

In pediatric patients with chronic functional constipation, one study showed that diaphragmatic breathing increased colonic persistalsis and improved the frequency of bowel movements.[7] The researchers believed this outcome was a direct result of the parasympathetic nervous system, which controls the rhythmic contractions of the intestines, being activated by the participants' breathing. Diaphragmatic breathing increases calmness and relaxation and brings you out of high-arousal states of mind. And your gut function can improve as a result. I find it so fascinating that something as "simple" as breathing can have such a powerful impact on the gut and body.

# BREATHWORK EXERCISES FOR THE GUT

While practicing any kind of breathwork can potentially benefit your gut, certain breathwork exercises and sequences will work better than others. Just like you would want health advice from a medical expert on your specific ailment, I prefer to use breathwork exercises designed by the pros that directly address the issues I'm dealing with.

Below, you'll find three breathwork exercises that improve gut health, courtesy of three stellar breathwork experts. I've also provided some background on each expert so you know who you're learning from. Please note that these are in no specific order, and you aren't expected to do them consecutively. I encourage you to try all of them in whatever order you'd like and see what works best for you!

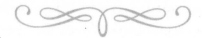

### 1. The Best Rest & Digest Breathwork Exercise for Beginners with Jesse Gros

*Jesse Gros is a life coach, author, and breathwork facilitator and teacher. Jesse has been teaching Pranayama breathwork for several years to groups as large as fifty as well as intimately one-on-one with clients. Jesse is the author of* The Freethinker's Guide to Coaching, My Life Coach Wears a Tutu, *and* Your Wild & Precious Life: Adventures in Conscious Creation. *Jesse leads transformational retreats all over the world through his retreat and coaching company, Insight Adventures. He holds a master's degree in spiritual psychology from the University of Santa Monica and is a Certified Life Coach, Breathwork Healer, and TED speaker coach. You can find Jesse on Instagram @jessegros or at InsightAdventures.com.*

Your mind will lie to you all day long if you let it. But the good news is, your body doesn't know how to lie. We see this truth reflected in popular culture. We say things like "Trust your gut," and "I had a gut feeling about it." The gut is the center of our emotional brain. It's also one of the key places our intuition communicates with us. Quite often, the problems we create for ourselves stem from not listening to this inner voice.

A breathwork client of mine who was feeling quite stuck in her life asked herself out loud one day in class, "When did I stop trusting my body?" What she was *really* asking was, "When did I hand over all of the control to my thinking mind?" How about you?

*How much do you trust your body? Do you follow your gut, or do you override it with rationality or dismissive thoughts?*

Many of our physical and emotional problems stem from not trusting the internal guidance our body is attempting to share with us every day. To move out of dysfunction and disorder, back into alignment with our natural state of health, we have to communicate directly with our body. One of the ways we do that is through **Pranayama breathwork**. This thousand-year-old technique activates your parasympathetic nervous system, calming your body and slowing activity in your prefrontal cortex, which in turn quiets that nagging, persistent voice in your head.

Sound too good to be true? I thought so at first. Well . . . with ten years of practice and teaching under my belt, I can tell you, it's worked magic for my clients and myself alike.

The breathing practice below is simple. You can do it in as little as fifteen minutes, and most folks I have worked with don't want to stop once they get going!

It involves two phases:

### Phase 1: Cleaning House

Most of us are not aware of how we take on other people's upset. Social media, the news, arguments with your loved ones, the guy on the freeway who cuts you off (and curses at you!) . . . all of these disturbances add up, putting you into a state of constant emotional defense. Once that armor is up, physical and emotional dysfunction set in.

This breathing technique is an emotional and psychic Roto-Rooter, cleaning out the upset that we accumulate throughout the day, and even unresolved baggage we have been carrying around for a long time.

### Phase 2: Receiving Gifts

Once we have cleared out stress and upset through the breath, we move into a calm space. There we can hear the messages our intuition or our "gut" has been attempting to communicate to us. These messages are gifts from our unconscious, directing us towards our authentic life path. Your body will respond with less stress and, quite often, improved gut function.

 ## The "Rest & Digest" Breathwork Exercise

*(Note: No experience or meditation skill necessary!)*

Set up your space so you won't be interrupted, and play some nice, relaxing music.

Lie on your back on a flat surface with your legs and arms flat at your sides, palms facing up, eyes closed. (It's best not to use a pillow, to keep your throat open.) Relax, and get ready to start the breathwork.

This is a three-part breath, all through the mouth (two breaths in, one breath out). Don't rush—do both inhalations and the exhalation at a speed that feels comfortable. Faster is not better; what matters most is keeping to a consistent rhythm throughout the exercise.

1. Breathe into your belly (your belly will rise).

2. Breath in the second breath and fill your upper chest (your chest rises).

3. Release and exhale all of the air.

**\*\*Repeat, continuing the three-part breath for at least 10–15 minutes.\*\***

In the beginning, you may notice that before your mind calms down, it may speed up with thoughts like, *Am I doing this right? Will this work for me? Why am I doing this?!* If this happens, just thank your mind for the feedback, and stay with the breath.

You may notice some tingling or a bit of dizziness in the very beginning.‡ That's normal; just stay with the breath at a nice, even, calm pace. If you find yourself

---

‡ You should not do the three-part breath without supervision if you are pregnant, have been diagnosed with heart disease, or have a history of a severe mental health disorder.

speeding up, just slow the breath back down. It doesn't have to be fast to be effective. Do what feels and comes naturally. Remember, you are in charge and can stop at any time.

You may also notice your hands tingling or feeling heavy. If that happens, switching to gentle nose breathing for a few minutes will restore normal feeling in your hands. Once you feel comfortable again, you can resume the three-part breath.

Try to set aside at least ten to fifteen minutes for this exercise, but you are also welcome to go longer if desired. I've led group sessions that have lasted as long as an hour.

## Bonus Step: Set Intentions

This work aligns very well with setting intentions. I like to think of intentions as giving your mind something to chew on. My favorite intention for breathwork:

> *I am open to the experience;*
> *I am open to receive; just let go.*

Repeat this in your mind for the first couple of minutes of the practice.

- - - - - - - - - - - - - - - - - - - - - - - - - - - - - - - - - - - - - - - - - - - - - - -

## 2. Breathwork for Better Digestion with Sachin Patel

*Sachin Patel is a father, husband, philanthropist, functional medicine practice success coach, speaker, author, breathwork facilitator, and plant medicine advocate. He believes that "the doctor of the future is the patient," and has committed himself to helping others raise their consciousness, activate their inner doctor, and initiate their deepest healing through the use of lifestyle and breathwork. Sachin founded the Living Proof Institute, through which he is pioneering a revolutionary approach to patient-centered healthcare. You can find Sachin on Instagram @thesachinpatel or at TheLivingProofInstitute.com/sachin-patel.*

Every single breath that we take matters. However, when it comes to digestion, how we breathe matters more than we might think, because the breath is the bridge between a sympathetic state and a parasympathetic state.

It's in our parasympathetic state that digestive function is optimized. In this state, blood flow is directed at the abdominal organs instead of the arms and legs. This enables us to improve stomach acid and enzyme production, enhance nutrient absorption, optimize bowel peristalsis, and upgrade detoxification through the liver and kidneys.

There are four keys to healthy digestive function that we want to pay attention to:

**Choose:** Choose the right foods to eat in the right amount at the right time of day.

**Chew:** Chew your food thoroughly to maximize digestion and absorption of nutrients.

**Chill:** Use your breath as a tool to shift your autonomic nervous system into a state of "rest and digest."

**Cherish:** Express gratitude for the meal you are about to eat to further enhance the parasympathetic state.

Sending blood (which is full of nutrients and oxygen) to the gut is critical for it to function properly, and it's essential that we do whatever we can to ensure we are enabling that. It's also critical to note that the digestive process does not stop after we've taken our last bite. That food will take hours to digest. Therefore, it's important to consider your internal state for several hours after you eat. This means you're working against yourself if you're relaxed *only* while you're eating and then jump right back into a stressful day. It's critical to digestive wellness that you are aware of how you manage your stress response once the food is in your body, too.

Breathwork is one of the most powerful relaxation tools that we have. The correct breathing techniques can induce an optimal state for digesting and assimilating your food, allowing you better access to the nutrition your food can provide. I'd like to offer some very practical breathing strategies that can help you get into the relaxed state that will let you best digest the delicious meals in this book and help you nourish your body before, during, and after you eat.

I've included two state-shifting breathing techniques to choose from for before you eat, based on your stress level, plus techniques designed to be used while eating and after eating/between meals. All should be done in a seated position.

. . . . . . . . . . . . . . . . . . . . . . . . . . . . . . . . . . . . . . . . . . . . . . . . . . . . .

## Breathing before Eating (choose one of the following)

### 1. Physiological sigh (when pre-meal stress is high)

1. Sit up nice and straight.

2. Play some relaxing music if possible.

3. Breathing through your nose, take a deep breath in.

4. At the very top of your breath, take another sharp breath in and hold for four seconds.

5. Release the breath through the mouth with a sigh—"ahhhhhhhh"—as you relax your shoulders and fully exhale.

6. Repeat four times.

7. Check in with yourself and where your stress levels are. If still high, repeat the exercise.

### 2. Box breathing (when pre-meal stress is low to moderate)

1. Sit up nice and straight.

2. Play some relaxing music if possible.

3. Breathe in through the nose for a count of four.

4. Hold for a count of four.

5. Exhale through the nose for a count of four.

6. Hold for a count of four.

7. Repeat steps 3–6 until your song is over.

## Breathing while Eating

1. Keep your mouth closed and breathe through your nose while you chew, so you can better taste and digest your food.

2. Breathe in for two to four seconds, and then slowly release your breath through the nose as you chew each bite, keeping your breathing calm and relaxed. The longer the exhale, the more your parasympathetic system will be activated.

## Breathing after Eating & Between Meals (wait at least two hours after eating)[‡]

1. Breathe through your nose as much as possible throughout the day.

2. As you breathe, your tongue should sit gently at the roof of your mouth to relax your jaw muscles.

3. Inhale for six seconds and exhale for six seconds as your breathing cadence.

4. Your breathing should be soft and undetectable to the person sitting next to you.

## 3. The 2X Breath Technique for Stress Reduction with Emily Fletcher

*Emily Fletcher is the founder of Ziva Meditation and the leading expert in meditation for performance. She has taught more than 40,000 people the skill of meditation. She is an international speaker and author. Her bestselling book,* Stress Less, Accomplish More, *debuted at #7 out of all books on Amazon and has been translated into twelve languages. You can find Emily on Instagram @emilystellafletcher or at ZivaMeditation.com.*

---

[‡] By this time, your digesting food will have moved from the stomach to the small intestine, clearing more space for breathwork. This may take longer if you have slow digestion or gastroparesis.

When we are dealing with big demands in our lives, a primitive part of the brain takes over. We've all been there. In such overwhelm, even though we know how we "should" be acting, our bodies simply don't want to listen. This is because you can't negotiate with your stress. When you are in fight-or-flight mode, not only does digestion shut down, but the *amygdala* (the fear center of the brain) takes over. The **amygdala** is an ancient, preverbal part of the brain. This is why "telling" yourself to relax when you're in a hyped-up stress moment (or worse, when someone else tells you to "just relax") doesn't work for many people. The part of you that is stressed doesn't understand language. It only understands pleasure and pain.

So instead of reasoning with your fear or stress, you have to shift the body physically and chemically. That is what the **2X breath technique** below will do for you.

This simple but powerful technique can keep you from spiraling into a cesspool of stress and help you become more present in the current moment. It also moves you from fight-or-flight into rest-and-digest, meaning that, over time, and especially if you do this before meals, you will start to see better gut health and easier digestion.

Don't let the 2X breath technique's simplicity fool you. The most profound truths are usually the simplest. And if you are on the edge of an anxiety attack, you don't need a complicated tool. You need something simple.

The magic is in doubling the length of the exhale. This calms the vagus nerve. Also, as vagal tone improves, information can start to flow from your gut to your brain and vice versa, opening you up to solutions from your second brain—the gut, your intuitive center.

Before starting any exercise, it is a good habit to check in with yourself and see how you are feeling. What is your set point? Where is stress being held in your body right now? Then you can celebrate your successes on the other side. Let's begin!

## The 2X Breath Technique

This exercise can be done sitting in a chair, with feet flat on the floor and eyes closed, or while walking. If you are feeling quite stressed and it is hard to sit still, then I recommend you start with walking, and transition to a seated position once you feel calmer.

1. Start by inhaling through your nose for two counts. Then exhale through your mouth for four counts. On the exhale, you can let the shape of your mouth be easy and the breath flow softly—no need to vocalize or create tension in your lips. If you are walking, try to match your breath to your steps by inhaling for two steps and exhaling for four steps.

2. Repeat. Inhale through your nose for two; exhale through your mouth for four. Keep doing this. Continue for about three minutes or fifteen breath cycles. As you repeat these cycles, you will find yourself connecting more with your body and your intuitive gut center as your mind quiets down.

3. Once you are fully back in your body and the "right now," think of three things you are most grateful for in this moment. No, really. List them on a sheet of paper or in a gratitude journal. It is impossible to be in both a stressful state *and* a state of gratitude at the same time. One emotion makes the other more subtle. And then it evaporates it.

Take note of how you were feeling before and how you feel afterwards. Give yourself a big internal high-five, and go about your day knowing there is power and integrity in tending to your gut health through your mental fitness.

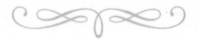

I've provided three exercises above, but to be clear: You don't have to do every one of these exercises to see results. Instead, try each one at your convenience and see which one or ones resonate with you. Like yoga or meditation, the practice of breathwork is deeply personal, and when you're starting out, it's all about figuring out what's most beneficial for you in each moment. And that can change over time, so be sure to come back to this chapter as you progress through your gut-healing journey and try these breathwork exercises again.

For more helpful resources and recordings of these breathwork exercises, visit **GutSMART Protocol.com**.

## Takeaways

Breathwork calms the nervous system and establishes the foundation upon which to build your mindfulness and meditation practices. But before you move on to the next chapter for some mindfulness practices and meditations that are sure to enhance your gut-healing results, let's take one more look at this chapter's main points. Then let's keep the momentum going!

1. The term *breathwork* refers to breathing exercises that employ *diaphragmatic breathing* (or deep breathing, discussed in chapter 10).

2. Diaphragmatic breathing involves breathing with the diaphragm. It is healthier than chest breathing, which most of us have been conditioned to do as a result of our hectic, rushed lifestyles or to maintain the illusion of a thin waist.

3. Because diaphragmatic breathing is so effective at lowering stress and switching on the parasympathetic nervous system, it has the potential to turbocharge your gut-healing results.

4. Breathing patterns tend to reflect our emotions. But the breath is also a way to change how our body and mind are feeling and, through that, our digestion.

5. When we are in fight-or-flight mode, digestion shuts down. When we breathe our way to a calm, relaxed state, it allows for easier digestion.

6. Breathwork is deeply personal. Try different exercises, and choose the one or ones that work best for you at any given moment. Revisit them every so often because you may find that one that didn't work for you before is the perfect fit for what you're going through now.

Chapter 12

---

# THE ZEN GUT: MEDITATIONS & MINDFULNESS FOR A HAPPY GUT

> *"You cannot have a happy gut without a calm mind and calm heart."*
>
> —Dr. Vincent Pedre

**You've made it to the final chapter in "Turbocharging Your Results,"** where we're going to dive into meditation and mindfulness. I've strategically placed this chapter after the breathwork chapter because, as I mentioned before, the two practices go hand in hand. I once heard a meditation teacher say, "I breathe in order to meditate." Meditation builds on the foundation you've laid down by practicing the previous chapter's breathwork exercises. And breathwork and meditation are two of the strongest tools you have to get you into a state of **mindfulness**, where you are calmly aware of the present moment. When you can get your mind to that place of Zen, your gut won't be far behind.

Like breathwork, meditation is not a new practice. The earliest records of meditation we have are from 1500 BCE,[1] but some archeologists date meditation back to 5000 BCE.[2] That means that meditation may be over 7,000 years old—wild to think about, right?—and only now are we starting to understand the science behind it and (here in the Western world) acknowledge its power. Multiple studies have shown that meditation benefits gut health, including for individuals suffering from IBS, by activating the vagus nerve. And a scientific literature review confirming that stress states disturb the gut microbiota, leading to dysbiosis and inflammation, also showed that meditation, by regulating the stress response, promotes a healthy gut flora that suppresses chronic inflammation and helps maintain a healthy gut lining.[3] It's taken us a while to recognize all of this . . . so let's not waste another second.

In this chapter, I'll give you a brief overview of meditation: how it's defined and what it means to meditate, what mindfulness is, the research on meditation, and of course, how meditation can improve your gut health. I've also included three written meditations—two from my absolute favorite meditation teachers and one from none other than *me*—all of which are geared toward boosting your gut health. (You can find recordings of these at **GutSMARTProtocol.com**.) By the end of the chapter, you will have a solid grasp of why meditation matters for gut health, and you'll have the guidance and resources you need to practice meditation on your own.

## WHAT ARE MEDITATION AND MINDFULNESS?

In the not-too-distant past, we may have thought of meditation as a yogi with a turban sitting on a mountain somewhere meditating—not something for regular people. Even in 1995, when I started meditating at the age of twenty-one, I kept it a secret from my medical school classmates, afraid I would be judged as the "weird" guy doing that "hippie thing." Instead, I became known as the "Zen" guy, and later on, the "Zen doctor." In the last few decades, meditation has become a widespread practice. And today, books on the power of mindfulness and meditation by *New York Times* bestselling authors like Deepak Chopra and Gabby Bernstein top the bestseller lists.

According to the National Center for Complementary and Integrative Health:

**Meditation** *is a mind and body practice that has a long history of use for increasing calmness and physical relaxation, improving psychological balance, coping with illness, and enhancing overall health and well-being.*[4]

While we typically think of meditating as sitting still and breathing deeply, there are many ways to enter *a meditative* or *mindful state*. As an example, if you are an artist, practicing your craft—painting, sculpting, or writing—could put you in a meditative state. The same goes for people who love exercise—you'll often hear runners say that running is meditative for them, and the same goes for yogis, cyclists, and other athletes who get *into the zone*. Even everyday behaviors like reading, going for long walks, or listening to music can be considered meditative because they can help you get out of your head and into your body. So, what kind of meditation are we talking about here in this chapter?

Meditation can look different for different people, but the feeling it gives every person is the same. It allows you to access a feeling of *mindfulness*—which is defined as being completely aware of the present moment, of all that's happening around you, and everything going on inside you.[5] We often hear people say that we should "live in the present," and what they mean is that we should practice mindfulness. Mindfulness and meditation are closely related and symbiotic: **Mindfulness improves our meditation, while meditation expands our mindfulness.**

. . . . . . . . . . . . . . . . . . . . . . . . . . . . . . . . . . . . . . . . . . . . . . . . . . . . . . . .

## Mindfulness is the basic human ability to be fully present, aware of where we are and what we're doing, and not overly reactive or overwhelmed by what's going on around us.[6]

. . . . . . . . . . . . . . . . . . . . . . . . . . . . . . . . . . . . . . . . . . . . . . . . . . . . . . . .

Your path to this mindful, meditative state is unique to you. Activities that some people find enjoyable, others find frustrating. (We all know someone who doesn't like yoga, for instance. Much to my dismay, I've had patients who have told me it doesn't work for them.) For the sake of simplicity, the kind of meditation I'm referring to—and the exercises I've included in this chapter—focus on quiet presence and deep breathing as vehicles for relaxation.

These exercises all employ the deep, diaphragmatic breath that you learned and practiced in chapter 10. (*Make sure you've mastered it before moving along to the meditations.*) And similar to the breathwork exercises in chapter 11, these meditations focus on shifting your body from a stressed-out, overstimulated state where your sympathetic nervous system is activated to a more relaxed, parasympathetic state. As you'll recall, being in a parasympathetic state is crucial for optimal gut health because stress, anxiety, and constantly being in fight-or-flight mode inevitably lead to gastrointestinal issues (and more).

## HOW MEDITATION HELPS THE GUT

There's a growing body of research that underscores the immense benefits of meditation for a variety of physiological and psychological ailments, from pain and high blood pressure to insomnia, depression, and anxiety.[7] More relevant to this book (and your gut health journey), though, is the effect meditation can have on digestive conditions. In several studies, meditation has been shown to reduce the severity of symptoms that stem from digestive conditions, including IBS and ulcerative colitis.[8] And of course, meditation is ideal for alleviating stress.

As you've read in previous chapters, the gut is profoundly affected by stress. Stress can cause symptoms like bloating, constipation, abdominal pain, and more. Through diaphragmatic breathing, meditation lowers the heart rate and switches the body into a parasympathetic state, the preferred state for optimal gut health and digestion.[9]

One study performed jointly at New York University, the University of California at San Diego, and the Chopra Foundation summed up the gut-stress connection well:

> *Psychological stress typically triggers a fight-or-flight response . . . which ultimately disturbs the microbiota. In the absence of stress, a healthy microbiota produces short-chain fatty acids that exert anti-inflammatory and antitumor effects. During stress, an altered gut microbial population affects the [production] of neurotransmitters mediated by the microbiome and gut barrier function [that is, gut permeability].[10]*

Meditation, the study's authors go on to note, "helps regulate the stress response, thereby suppressing chronic inflammation states and maintaining a healthy gut barrier function."[11]

Bottom line: Decreasing your stress, whether through meditation or other means, is going to improve your gut health straight away. We cannot wash away our stress with meditation, but we *can* increase our adaptability and resilience to it so that it does not affect us in negative ways. And the best part is that you don't have to meditate for long to get the benefits.[12] Meditating for as little as ten minutes a day can have a noticeable impact on your overall health![13]

# MEDITATIONS & MINDFULNESS FOR THE GUT

To get you started, here are three guided meditations, written by Emily Fletcher (who you'll remember from the breathwork chapter), Amanda Gilbert, and me.

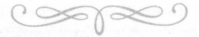

### 1. Go from Gut Stress to Gut Bliss with Emily Fletcher

When the body gets stressed, it launches into fight-or-flight mode. This sympathetic reaction can cause issues like excess acid production in the stomach. So if we are dealing with chronic stress, it can lead to chronic acidity in the digestive system, which leads to gut issues like inflammation and IBS. By using this and other meditation exercises, you are getting out of the sympathetic overdrive state and into the parasympathetic state—that is, you're getting out of fight-or-flight and into rest-and-digest.

I recommend doing this exercise as you read it the first time. Hear the words in your mind as if you are being guided in real time. Then read it again without practicing it. The goal is to commit it to memory so you can guide yourself through it on your own.

This is a great meditation to do to remind yourself of how much bliss you have already created in your life so you can return to that peaceful place even in the moments when things feel overwhelming.

## Stress-to-Bliss Meditation

1. To start, have a seat someplace where your back is supported and your head is free.

2. Close your eyes, and give yourself a moment to arrive, letting your body, your mind, and your spirit focus on the present—right here, right now.

3. Take a big, delicious inhale through your nose, and exhale through your mouth. We're going to inhale through the nose for the count of two, and exhale through the mouth for the count of four, just like you did in the *2x Breath* exercise I taught you in the previous chapter. Repeat four times: in for two, out for four.

4. Now, we're going to prolong the breath. Breathe in for four and out for eight. So inhale 2, 3, 4. And out through your mouth—exhale 2, 3, 4, 5, 6, 7, 8. In through your nose for four and out through your mouth for eight, all the way to empty. Then let that air flow back into your lungs—taking the biggest inhale you've taken all day, breathing all the way down into your belly. This time, as you exhale, soften your brow, soften your jaw, soften your shoulders, and open up your heart, relaxing the belly.

5. Next, inhale all the way down into your pelvis. Take the biggest inhale you've taken all year. And as you exhale, starting at the shoulders, let your shoulders hang soft, let your heart open, let your belly hang loose, feel the weight of your legs against the chair and your feet on the ground all the way down into the earth.

6. Now sit quietly, softly breathing, for three to five minutes, allowing whatever comes up in your mind to simply flow by. Don't hold on to your thoughts, just observe them as if you are looking at yourself from the outside. When you feel complete, move on to the next and final step.

7. Final breath: Inhale all the way down into your toes, and exhale fully. When you come to the bottom of this exhale, you can keep your eyes closed and let your breath be easy and natural, not elongating or forcing or controlling the breath in any direction. Enjoy the feeling of bliss this has created in your body, and let it resonate into your gut.

At the end of this meditation, I invite you to check in with yourself—your body, your mind, your heart, and your gut. How do you feel now versus how you felt when you started the exercise? Did you have a knot in your stomach? Did your abdominal muscles feel tense? How do you feel in your abdomen now? Take note of the changes you experience each time, and watch your gut health improve before your very eyes.

## 2. A Mindful Eating Ritual for Resting & Digesting with Amanda Gilbert

*Amanda Gilbert is a meditation teacher, lecturer of mindfulness at the University of Southern California, and the author of* Kindness Now: A 28-Day Guide to Living with Authenticity, Intention, and Compassion. *Amanda has conducted clinical research on the biological and psychological effects of mindfulness and meditation. Her formal meditation training has been with UCLA's Mindful Awareness Research Center, in Primordial Sound Meditation with Deepak Chopra, and within the Insight Meditation tradition at InsightLA. Amanda has led meditation for top companies like NBC, Paramount Pictures, W Hotels, Merrill Lynch, Macy's, and YouTube. You can find her at AmandaGilbert Meditation.com.*

Mindfulness is one of the few precious ways we have as human beings to consciously engage with rest and inner connection. It is a sacred sanctuary for learning not only more about ourselves, but also how best to support our mental and physical well-being by creating routines and rituals that assist our personal healing.

Making everyday tasks and moments, such as drinking your morning cup of coffee or strolling to work, into special rituals allows for the mundane actions of our daily lives to become chock-full of intention, mindfulness, and healing potential. By turning an ordinary breakfast or lunch break at work into an opportunity to slow down or pause, you start to support your mind-body-brain-gut well-being through self-care, just by bringing this type of special presence into your day-to-day life.

Mindful eating is a practice that primes your nervous system to arrive into a state of rest-and-digest. With mindful eating, mealtimes become a built-in moment of mindfulness, and snacking becomes sacred—a time to truly nourish body and mind, allowing the nutrients in your food to be fully assimilated, and a ritual that helps foster your intentions for a healthy gut.

I promise that if you follow the mindful eating ritual meditation I share below, you will notice your meal and snack times turning into a meaningful pause you look forward to. Restoring, honoring, and connecting with the food you are receiving creates the conditions for real healing. Rituals have been used for hundreds of years to bring intention and sacred connection to the mundane. Let your new three-part mindful eating ritual be a way to make each moment before, during, and after you eat the supportive restorative time you have been craving.

(*Note from Dr. Pedre: You can combine this ritual with the Breathwork for Better Digestion practices taught by Sachin Patel in chapter 11.*)

. . . . . . . . . . . . . . . . . . . . . . . . . . . . . . . . . . . . . . . . . . . . . . . . . . . . . . . .

## Your Pre-Meal Ritual

The moment you know you are about to take a bite of food is when your premeal ritual begins. Whether you're opening up a bag of seaweed snacks or sitting down for a five-course meal, prepare yourself for your mindful eating practice by pausing and intentionally slowing down.

1. Allow your eyes to close gently for a moment.

2. Feel the texture of the surface your hands are resting upon.

3. Invite in an internal moment of pause by taking a deep breath in . . . and out.

4. Set an intention for your eating time. For example, your intention can be one of these mindful eating mantras or phrases:
   "I give myself permission to slow down."
   "I allow my body to receive these nutrients in a state of rest."
   "I can feel good as my body properly digests."
   Or use whatever unique mantra feels most supportive to your body, gut, and mind right now.

## Mindful Eating Ritual

Once you've set your intention in your premeal ritual, start your mindful eating ritual. Remember, your mindful eating practice is a way of slowing down so your body is in a supportive state to improve digestion and assimilate the nutrients it is receiving.

1. With each bite of food, invite in the opportunity to slow down and enjoy your snack or meal.

2. Sense your hands or utensil bringing the bite of food to your mouth.

3. Explore the burst of flavors found within the first chew or two.

4. Eat each bite slowly. Chew each morsel of food thoroughly.

5. When you are ready to swallow your bite of food, bring your full attention to the food as it moves down the back of your throat and finds its way to your belly.

6. Pause now, and rest in the sacred recognition that you just took in the orchestra of nutrients, calories, and biodiversity, and that it is now meeting your community of gut flora and preparing to nourish your whole body.

7. Take a moment to appreciate how this one bite of food has contributed to the health and happiness of your body, mind, and gut.

8. Continue eating mindfully in this way until you notice your body reaching fullness and satiety.

## Your Post-Meal Ritual

To best ritualize your daily moments of eating, make sure to end each snack or meal with gratitude and reflection. Once you're done eating, take a moment to pause once again before you move into the rest of your day.

1. Close your eyes and thank all of the organisms, bacteria, humans, and elements from the natural world that were a part of your meal.

2. Feel your part in the interconnected web of eating, receiving, assimilating, and then giving back.

3. Take a deep breath in . . . and let it out of the body slowly.

4. When you are ready, slowly open your eyes.

Allow any feelings of rest, rejuvenation, and inner connection to carry with you into the rest of your day.

. . . . . . . . . . . . . . . . . . . . . . . . . . . . . . . . . . . . . . . . . . . . . . . . .

When you make your meals into a ritual and practice mindful eating, you will feel the digestive harmony in your body improving and your overall mood thriving. And this all happens just by slowing down and savoring each delicious bite, welcoming it in as part of your healing journey.

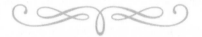

### 3. Dr. Pedre's Gut-Love Meditation

When your gut is constantly giving you trouble, it's easy to fall into an adversarial relationship with it. This meditation is designed to help you create more harmony with your gut so you can develop a new symbiotic relationship with the "cornerstone of your health." Set aside ten minutes to do this meditation. You can do it daily, but aim for at least three times per week while working on healing your digestive system.

#### Gut-Love Meditation

1. Get into a comfortable seated position in a chair with your feet flat on the floor or, alternatively, on the floor in lotus pose with your legs crossed, sitting on a cushion to support your pelvis and lower back.

2. Make sure your spine is erect and your shoulders are relaxed, falling away from your ears.

3. Close your eyes. Tune in to your breath. Breathe in. Breathe out. Soft and easy. Do this for one minute.

4. Now, bring your focus to your abdomen. Take a deep breath, breathing in through your nose with your diaphragm; take a pause for one second, then slowly breathe out through your nose, belly button toward your back, squeezing out as much air as possible. Just like in the 2X *Breath* in chapter 11, try to make your exhale twice as long as your inhale. Repeat this breath pattern for at least thirty seconds or until you feel you've fallen into a comfortable rhythm.

5. Next, expand the breath, breathing in for a count of four, followed by a one- to two-second pause, then breathing out for a count of eight.

6. While continuing this breath, place your hands one over the other on your belly button (middle belly). Bring your focus to where your hands are—your gut.

7. Think of gratitude. Thank your gut for breaking down the foods you eat and for providing the nutrients needed to nourish your brain and entire body.

8. Focus all that gratitude into your digestive system. Do this for at least four minutes.

9. Now transform that feeling of gratitude into unconditional love for your gut. Send the warmth of compassion and self-love to your gut. Feel that love spreading like the roots of a tree, reaching into every corner and crevice inside your digestive system.

10. Shower your internal organs of digestion and assimilation with that love, including your stomach, the small and large intestines, and your powerful detox organ—the liver.

11. Send love to the one hundred trillion microorganisms inside your gut that we call the microbiome. Let them know you appreciate the way they help your body care for itself.

12. Remember to breathe. Deep, diaphragmatic breaths.

13. Now expand that love, all of its warmth and compassion that is strongly rooted in your gut, to encase your whole body.

14. Bask in the feeling of love that is coming from your gut. Know that your gut-love consumes all of you now.

15. End by thanking your gut for being the foundation of holistic wellness for your entire body.

16. Place your hands on your lap.

17. Take a deep breath through your nose. Let it out through the mouth with a forceful exhalation. Repeat two more times.

18. Wiggle your toes. Wiggle your fingers. Open your eyes. Come back into mindful presence, becoming aware of your surroundings again.

Congratulations! You have completed your gut-love meditation. Feel the sense of inner peace it gives you. Know that each time you do this meditation, you increase the healing potential of your gut. You are turbocharging your results for better gut health and holistic wellness.

For additional helpful resources and recordings of these meditations and the breathwork exercises, visit **GutSMARTProtocol.com**.

## Takeaways

Once you master breathwork, the natural next step is to learn and practice mindfulness and meditation. Together, these form a powerful combination of tools to use to *turbocharge* your gut-healing results.

1.  Meditation has been around for thousands of years, and there's a growing body of evidence that meditation benefits gut health.

2.  Generally speaking, the goal of meditation is to increase mental calmness and physical relaxation.

3.  Meditation shifts the body from fight-or-flight into rest-and-digest, which is ideal for gut function and healing.

4.  Meditation can help ease symptoms of digestive conditions like IBS and ulcerative colitis. By lowering stress levels, it can also help with bloating, constipation, abdominal pain, and more.

5.  Meditation is like medicine for your heart, soul, and digestive system. Meditation cannot wash away your stress, but it *can* increase your adaptability and resilience to it so that it does not affect you in negative ways.

6.  Mindfulness when eating gifts us with the power to connect with the nutrients and food we are receiving, creating an internal state that makes real healing possible. By making your meals mindful and your snacks sacred, your body can assimilate the nutrients it needs more effectively.

7.  Meditation can be an incredible tool for creating more harmony with your gut.

8.  Sending your gut love is a powerful way to reframe your relationship with it (especially if that relationship has been antagonistic in the past) into a positive one that allows healing to happen.

# WHAT'S NEXT? LIVING THE GUTSMART LIFE

> *"Life is about finding your center. When it comes to your health, that center is your gut."*
>
> —Dr. Vincent Pedre

**If you've made it this far, you are, without question, a part of the** GutSMART community! You've now completed *The GutSMART Protocol*, and are well on your way to a happy gut for life. Seriously! Give yourself a pat on the back! You've been through a lot, and you're still standing because you never gave up. My hope is that reading this book and going through the 14-day protocol will give you an even stronger belief in your body's ability to heal beyond what you thought was possible.

Living a GutSMART life is not just about eating a healthy diet, following a specific program, or taking the right supplements (which I discuss in my book *Happy Gut: The Cleansing Program to Help You Lose Weight, Gain Energy, and Eliminate Pain*). It's about the choices you make every day that ultimately become a part of your lifestyle.

The truth is that striving for a GutSMART life is not a linear journey. Many obstacles can get in the way, especially when you're healing from years of poor dietary choices, antibiotics, chronic stress, and more. And no matter how much gut healing you do, you can still encounter roadblocks along the way. For example, you might need antibiotics for a dental procedure. Maybe you go through a stressful divorce, or have to deal with an unfriendly boss or the stress of aging parents. Who knows?! The point is that some things are unavoidable, and setbacks are to be expected.

My hope is that, regardless of the setbacks, I have helped you build not just a platform for your health (starting with your gut) but also a foundation of knowledge that will allow you to be your own health guru on your healing journey. This is about so much more than just your gut-centric symptoms, as you learned in chapter 1.

I want to offer you the opportunity to keep learning by signing up for my newsletter at **HappyGutLife.com**, where you can gain greater wisdom and more tools to help you heal and maintain a healthy gut.

---

### FREE GIVEAWAY: Top 10 Tips for a Healthy, Happy Gut

Speaking of tools, I have a gift for you! I believe in rewarding those who do the work. So, I'd love to share with you my *Top 10 Tips for a Healthy, Happy Gut*, which summarizes much of the wisdom found in this book as well as in *Happy Gut*. In it, I share my top ten strategies to achieve bloat-free, easy digestion and have boundless energy, greater mental clarity, and effortless weight loss, even without counting calories. Simply go to **HappyGutLife.com/top10tips** to download your **free copy** today.

---

Take what you have learned in this book, along with my free guide, and use them to foster your intuitive inner-knowing of which foods do and do not work for you. Because if there is just one piece of advice I can leave you with, it's this:

## Learn to trust your gut intuition—that inner voice guiding you to make the right food choices.

The knowledge and self-understanding you've gained from reading *The Gut-SMART Protocol*, completing the GutSMART Quiz, and doing the breathwork and meditation exercises, along with the experience you've gained from following the 14-day protocol in this book, have all strengthened your ability to listen to that inner intuitive voice.

Living GutSMART with a happy gut is ultimately about listening to your body. Our bodies are constantly trying to communicate with us, and through the vagus nerve (remember chapter 10), your gut is sending a lot of signals up to your brain. Make time to quiet yourself enough to stop and listen. Trust it. And if you need help listening better, flip back to Part IV, "Turbocharging Your Results," and try practicing the meditation and breathing exercises again.

I have more to share with you in the Appendix about how you can deepen your results from *The GutSMART Protocol*. In the meantime, I love hearing from my readers. Come follow me on Instagram **@drpedre** and let me know how your experience with this book has been.

We all have the potential to be healers, for ourselves and for each other. Your voice is important, and it can help others find their way to their own gut healing as well as help me serve people better. I'd love your candid feedback on what you liked and what you would want me to change or improve. Together, we can have the greatest positive impact on people's health, because the healthier we become as a community, the healthier we can be as individuals. When we as a society have greater faith in and adherence to healthy living, it takes much less energy for each of us to live a healthy lifestyle. We tend to forget how powerful we are—when acting collectively we can change the fabric of our culture and improve our combined wellness.

So here's my ask: Take your experience of reading and following *The Gut-SMART Protocol* and share it by leaving an honest review on Amazon. Don't hold anything back, because your words can help others find their way to their own healing.

And here's my gratitude: Thank you for making it to the end of *The GutSMART Protocol*. You are a true wellness warrior! I applaud you! And with these tools, you are well on your way to healing your gut, transforming your health, living your best life ever, and making a positive impact on healing the world. Give yourself a big hug of self-love. You are part of a movement to make the entire planet a healthier place for everyone.

I hope this book continues to serve you in unexpected ways, peeling away the layers of gut-related health problems needed to fully actualize your well-being, so that you, and I, and everyone who benefits from this book can show up in the world as the best versions of ourselves.

Again, I congratulate you on your commitment to yourself! Keep it going, and never lose faith that with enough time, dedication, and a positive mental attitude, a happy gut and total healing are within reach and can be yours for a lifetime.

Appendix

# HOW TO TAKE YOUR GUT HEALING ONE STEP FURTHER

## (+ A Special Offer for *The GutSMART Protocol* Readers)

While I wrote this book to be as comprehensive as possible and know that the protocol will make a major difference in building your foundation of well-being, some of you may need to go beyond it to level up your gut health. Once you've completed the 14-day GutSMART Protocol (perhaps more than once), you may be wondering if there's a **next step** you can take?

At this point, you've seen what a program like the GutSMART Protocol can do for your gut health, but maybe you're still dealing with some lingering gut issues or gut-related symptoms you've identified by reading this book. Or maybe you loved the GutSMART Protocol so much, and it worked so well for you, that you don't want it to end—you want to deepen your healing! In either case, a longer, more extensive program may be what you need to get you feeling your absolute best—the best you've felt in years, the best you could ever feel. The most common question I get is, "What should I do next?" For you, I have a post-protocol recommendation: the HAPPY GUT® REBOOT: 28-Day Cleanse.

# WHAT YOU CAN EXPECT

Because the HAPPY GUT® REBOOT 28-Day Cleanse is a more thorough, deep-healing program, the transformation you can expect to see upon completing it may be even greater than what you've seen from the GutSMART Protocol.

By the end of the REBOOT, you will have:

- shed unwanted pounds from your waist (without counting calories!)
- removed gut irritants and toxins from your body
- repaired your gut lining
- bid farewell to bloating for good
- made heartburn a thing of the past
- improved your health from the inside out
- regained boundless energy (seriously, you won't know what to do with it all!)
- balanced your hormones (no more mood swings!)
- prevented or turned back the clock on autoimmune disease
- drastically lowered your stress and anxiety levels
- optimized your focus and mental clarity

And on top of all that, you'll be glowing from the inside out. People who complete the 28-day cleanse always tell me that *everything about them feels brighter*—their skin, complexion, overall mood, energy levels . . . everything. This program will give you a sense of security, contentment, and well-being like you've never known, and in doing so, it will boost your confidence and self-esteem.

Wondering if this program is right for you? Here's what people like you had to say after completing the HAPPY GUT® REBOOT 28-Day Cleanse:

> *I was sick, tired, and anxious, and felt like I was not myself physically or mentally at all. After the 28-Day Happy Gut Cleanse, I had* **constant all-day energy** *(with NO coffee at all anymore!) and no afternoon crash, and I* **felt calmer**, *more centered, and* **more focused** *than I've been in a very long time. I now* **sleep better** *than I ever have and* **wake up easier** *than before.*
>
> *—Kathy M.*

*If you've suffered from chronic issues for a while and want to feel better and get healthier, **twenty-eight days is nothing compared to however long you have been suffering**. I was experiencing a lot of skin issues. After the cleanse, my hives and rashes are gone, and my rosacea has disappeared.*

*—Mavic C.*

*My healing reached an entirely different level when I participated in the Happy Gut Cleanse.*

*As a business owner, I spend a lot of time with clients, and that requires a lot of energy. I was traveling a lot and got caught in a loop of jet lag, sleep deprivation, and poor eating habits. I love my work and wanted to serve more people, but I was on the verge of burnout. Dr. Pedre suggested the Happy Gut Cleanse to reset my metabolism and release unwanted weight. **The program was easy to follow, with clear step-by-step instructions and simple, delicious recipes that were fun to eat and fun to prepare.***

*I **effortlessly lost eleven pounds eating foods I love**, and I was never hungry! I **had consistent, sustainable energy**. I reignited my passion for my work. I **slept soundly every night** and woke up before my alarm, raring to go every morning. I **now know intuitively what my body needs most and can care for myself at higher levels than ever before**. Thank you, Dr. Pedre!*

*—Lee W.*

## HOW TO START YOUR TOTAL TRANSFORMATION

If the above speaks to you, then the HAPPY GUT® REBOOT 28-Day Cleanse is the next step in your gut healing! It's a complete gut reboot, and while it's longer than the GutSMART Protocol, I've taken all the roadblocks out of your way. It is *designed to be completed*. In other words, no matter what your personal obstacles are—lack of discipline, lack of time, indecision from information overload, or trouble committing and sticking to programs—the REBOOT addresses them and gives you the tools to overcome them. Plus, now that you've done two weeks with the GutSMART Protocol, I can assure you that twenty-eight days will feel like a breeze!

The cleanse is a proven, doctor-created solution that can help you reverse or prevent chronic disease, lose weight, and improve much more than just your gut health. It's backed by twenty years of research and thousands of success stories. I can't stress it enough: You cannot go wrong with this program.

The HAPPY GUT® REBOOT 28-Day Cleanse is for you if:

- You've been feeling tired, mentally foggy, and bloated, and are looking for a way to reboot your health in a way that is easy to do.
- You are ready to put an end for good to an irritated stomach and suffering from things like heartburn, diarrhea, and constipation.
- You are tired of calorie-counting diets with boring recipes that yield mediocre results.
- You want to get through the workday without having to drink that second, third, or fourth cup of coffee and still feel full of energy at the end of the day.
- You want to wake up and jump out of bed, ready to take on the day.
- You're on your gut health journey and are looking for the next best step!

## A SPECIAL OFFER FOR GUTSMART PROTOCOL READERS

As a thank-you for reading this book and trusting the process, I'm offering all *GutSMART Protocol* readers a special discount on the HAPPY GUT® REBOOT 28-Day Cleanse. Go to **GutSMARTProtocol.com/happygut** to claim your discount today! You won't find this discount anywhere else. It's my deepest discount, and it's just for you as a *thank-you* for saying YES! to getting GutSMART.

The HAPPY GUT® REBOOT is a bridge to a new, healthier version of you. I hope you'll give it a chance to show you how it can transform your health and life for the better, just like it did for Audrey:

*By day three of the cleanse, **my reflux was GONE**. And it hasn't returned. **I lost inches on my waist** and am **no longer bloated**. My digestion is normal. I don't have diarrhea, constipation, or cramps. It's amazing!*

Yours in gut health,

*Dr. Pedre*

AMERICA'S GUT DR.

# ACKNOWLEDGMENTS

**A book is a collaborative work of art that could not possibly come** into being without the shared vision and intention of a team of extraordinary people. I am grateful for so many people who either had a direct hand in creating this book or have provided the support that has allowed me to expand, dream, and envision how I can better help people.

My son, Ambrose: You bring meaning and completeness to my life. Thank you for your love, your compassion, and our shared silly moments of laughter. My sister Lisi: You are my rock when I most need support. My sister Laura: You are bottled happiness that brings a smile to my face.

My team: Jackie, your care and support of our patients allows me to spend more time in my zone of genius. Thank you for providing peace of mind that all is taken care of while I wear my many hats. And José, COO of Happy Gut Life, you are the right hand to my left hand, balancing my abstract creative mind with the fine-tuned precision of a virtuoso musician. Thank you for pushing me to be more authentically, lovingly myself in all the work I do.

My patients: Thank you for entrusting me with your care. Many of you were almost ready to give up when we met, and I am truly honored to have been a part of your wellness journey. You serve as my inspiration to evolve, improve, and expand from helping the ones in my practice to guiding the many I may never meet in person.

My literary agent, Stephany Evans: It was your "yes" when I was an unknown, soon-to-be author that has gifted me with the ability to have a huge impact on the health of the world. The greatest gift you gave me was seeing my potential and providing the guidance I needed to harness what was waiting to be put into words for the benefit of thousands.

Glenn, Leah, Claire, Adrienne, Sarah, Kim, Lindsay, and the rest of my team at BenBella Books: Your enthusiasm, kindness, and guidance has gracefully helped breathe life into the proposal that became this book. Thank you for also seeing the vision, believing in me, and providing the detailed support needed to bring this book to all the people who desperately need it. Working with you has felt like coming home.

More words for my editor, Leah: I am eternally grateful for the love and support you poured into this book in time, edits, and comments that helped me sharpen the message and make it as crystal clear and understandable as possible for the readers.

Ray, my writing and research assistant: Thank you for your can-do attitude and openness to feedback, and for putting your love and energy into this book. Working with you was a breath of fresh air.

Candace Johnson, my collaborative editor: From *Happy Gut* to *GutSMART*, we have now worked together over a span of two books. Your attention to detail, indefatigable ability to review each chapter over and over as we refined them (*and never complain*), and honest feedback have been welcome friends that have allowed this book to come to fruition with ease and grace.

Chef Lee Holmes: You made creating the recipes and meal plans for this book a breeze. You are one of my soul sisters, and I appreciate you so much for putting your heart into the fabulous and creative recipes, even with the challenge of keeping to the restrictions of each GutSMART Score category, while adding color and variety to this protocol. You've shown once again that eating for gut health never has to be boring!

Summer Bock, the Fermentationist: Your input on fermented foods—when to use them and how much to start with—was greatly appreciated, as are all of our nerdy science discussions. You have been a great sounding board for this book.

Registered dietician and integrative nutritionist Eleni Ottalagana: Thank you for your expert input on categorizing foods in the GutSMART food list.

Our breathwork and meditation gurus, Jesse Gros, Lee Holden, Emily Fletcher, Sachin Patel, and Amanda Gilbert: You are all truly spiritual ninjas. Thank you for your contributions to this book.

My food photo team, food photographer Andreana Bitsis and food stylist Eidia Moni: Wow! There is one word to describe how working with you two on the photographs for the recipes in this book felt—it was FLOW. From the preproduction to working tirelessly during a jam-packed three-day weekend of dawn-to-dusk cooking, setting, and photographing to the postproduction editing, you made what felt like a daunting task fun and dynamic. Thank you for bringing my vision for the recipes to life in a way that exceeded my greatest expectations.

My multitalented graphic designer, Eidia, who also did the food styling: Thank you for helping put the abstract ideas in my head into simple, engaging graphics that visually capture, explain, and enhance the concepts in this book. You did an amazing job!

My social media and PR team, Theresa, Bonnie, and Jade: Thank you for helping me put my message out there in an attention-grabbing way.

Dr. David Perlmutter: I am immensely grateful to you for your support throughout the years. Thank you for writing the foreword to this book when it was merely in its infancy.

Dr. Mark Hyman, Deepak Chopra, Dr. Andrew Weil, JJ Virgin, Dr. Joe Dispenza, Dr. Kellyann Petrucci, Dr. Patrick Hanaway, and the list goes on: Thank you for your courage to be voices of change, your desire to help others, and the trails you have blazed that I have humbly used as inspiration to become a change agent in wellness, just like all of you.

Finally, thank you to my functional medicine family, all of the inspirational healthpreneurs, influencers, and worldwide health warriors I've come to know, and the innumerable people who are part of my extended soul family: Keep spreading the word and shining bright!

# SCIENTIFIC CITATIONS

## Introduction

1   United Nations Department of Economic and Social Affairs, Population Division (2022). World Population Prospects 2022: Summary of Results. UN DESA/POP/2022/TR/NO. 3.

2   Lovell, R. M., & Ford, A. C. (2012, July). Global prevalence of and risk factors for irritable bowel syndrome: A meta-analysis. *Clinical Gastroenterology and Hepatology*, 10(7), 712–721. https://doi.org/10.1016/j.cgh.2012.02.029

3   Davis, C. D. (2016, July–August). The gut microbiome and its role in obesity. *Nutrition Today*, 51(4), 167–174. https://doi.org/10.1097/NT.0000000000000167

4   Boutagy, N. E., McMillan, R. P., Frisard, M. I., & Hulver, M. W. (2016, May). Metabolic endotoxemia with obesity: Is it real and is it relevant? *Biochimie, 124,* 11–20. https://doi.org/10.1016/j.biochi.2015.06.020

## Chapter 1

1   Harvard Health Publishing. (2021, April 1). *Feed your gut.* Harvard Health Publishing/Harvard Medical School. https://www.health.harvard.edu/staying-healthy/feed-your-gut

2   UNESCO. (2012, November 20). *Ocean life: The marine age of discovery.* UNESCO. https://en.unesco.org/news/ocean-life-marine-age-discovery-0

3   National Geographic Society. (n.d.). *Biodiversity.* https://www.nationalgeographic.org/encyclopedia/biodiversity

4   Langdon, A., Crook, N., & Dantas, G. (2016, April 13). The effects of antibiotics on the microbiome throughout development and alternative approaches for therapeutic modulation. *Genome Medicine, 8*(39). https://doi.org/10.1186/s13073-016-0294-z

5   Paradis, T., Bègue, H., Basmaciyan, L., Dalle, F., & Bon, F. (2021, March 2). Tight junctions as a key for pathogens invasion in intestinal epithelial cells. *International Journal of Molecular Sciences, 22*(5), 2506. https://doi.org/10.3390/ijms22052506

6    Ghoshal, U. C., Shukla, R., & Ghoshal, U. (2017). Small intestinal bacterial overgrowth and irritable bowel syndrome: A bridge between functional organic dichotomy. *Gut Liver, 11*(2), 196–208. https://doi.org/10.5009/gnl16126

7    Lovell, R. M., & Ford, A. C. (2012, July 1). Global prevalence of and risk factors for irritable bowel syndrome: A meta-analysis. *Clinical Gastroenterology and Hepatology, 10*(7), 712–721. https://doi.org/10.1016/j.cgh.2012.02.029

8    Institute for Quality and Efficiency in Health Care (IQWiG). (2010, November). What is an inflammation? *Informed Health Online* [Internet]. https://www.ncbi.nlm.nih.gov/books/NBK279298/

9    Damnjanović, Z., Jovanović, M., Nagorni, A., Radojković, M., Sokolović, D., Damnjanović, G., Đinđić, B., Smiljković, I., Kamenov, A., & Damnjanović, I. (2013, February). Correlation of inflammation parameters and biochemical markers of cholestasis with the intensity of lipid peroxidation in patients with choledocholithiasis. *Vojnosanitetski Pregled, 70*(2) 170–176. https://doi.org/10.2298/VSP1302170D

10   Vighi, G., Marcucci, F., Sensi, L., Di Cara, G., & Frati, F. (2008, September). Allergy and the gastrointestinal system. *Clinical and Experimental Immunology, 153, Suppl 1,* 3–6. https://doi.org/10.1111/j.1365-2249.2008.03713.x

11   Mu, Q., Kirby, J., Reilly, C. M., & Luo, X. M. (2017, May 23). Leaky gut as a danger signal for autoimmune diseases. *Frontiers in Immunology, 8.* https://doi.org/10.3389/fimmu.2017.00598

12   Paray, B. A., Albeshr, M. F., Jan, A. T., & Rather, I. A. (2020, December 21). Leaky gut and autoimmunity: An intricate balance in individuals health and the diseased state. *International Journal of Molecular Science, 21*(24), 9770. https://doi.org/10.3390/ijms21249770

13   Lens-Pechakova, L. S. (2019, November 10). Centenarian rates and life expectancy related to the death rates of multiple sclerosis, asthma, and rheumatoid arthritis and the incidence of type 1 diabetes in children. *Rejuvenation Research, 19*(1), 53–58. https://doi.org/10.1089/rej.2015.1690

## Chapter 2

1    Salem, I., Ramser, A., Isham, N., & Ghannoum, M. A. (2018, July 10). The gut microbiome as a major regulator of the gut-skin axis. *Frontiers in Microbiology, 9,* 1459. https://doi.org/10.3389/fmicb.2018.01459

2    Clark, A. K., Haas, K. N., & Sivamani, R. K. (2017, May). Edible plants and their influence on the gut microbiome and acne. *International Journal of Molecular Science, 18*(5), 1070. https://doi.org/10.3390/ijms18051070

3    Foster, J. A., Rinaman, L., & Cryan, J. F. (2017, March 19). Stress & the gut-brain axis: Regulation by the microbiome. *Neurobiology of Stress, 7,* 124–136. https://doi.org/10.1016/j.ynstr.2017.03.001

4    Salem et al. 2018.

5    Salem et al. 2018.

6   Bowe, W. P., & Logan, A. C. (2011). Acne vulgaris, probiotics and the gut-brain-skin axis—back to the future? *Gut Pathogens*, 3(1), 1. https://doi.org/10.1186/1757-4749-3-1

7   Gravina, A. G., Federico, A., Ruocco, E., Lo Schiavo, A., Masarone, M., Tuccillo, C., Peccerillo, F., Miranda, A., Romano, L., de Sio, C., de Sio, I., Persico, M., Ruocco, V., Riegler, G., Loguercio, C., & Romano, M. (2015). *Helicobacter pylori* infection but not small intestinal bacterial overgrowth may play a pathogenic role in rosacea. *United European Gastroenterology Journal*, 3(1), 17–24. https://doi.org/10.1177/2050640614559262

8   Salem et al. 2018.

9   Salem et al. 2018.

10  Dagnelie, M. A., Montassier, E., Khammari, A., Mounier, C., Corvec, S., & Dréno, B. Inflammatory skin is associated with changes in the skin microbiota composition on the back of severe acne patients. *Experimental Dermatology*, 28(8), 961–967. https://doi.org/10.1111/exd.13988

11  Dréno, B., Dagnelie, M. A., Khammari, A., & Coverc, S. (2020, September 10). The skin microbiome: A new actor in inflammatory acne. *American Journal of Clinical Dermatology* 21, 18–24. https://doi.org/10.1007/s40257-020-00531-1

12  Yan, H.-M., Zhao, H.-J., Guo, D.-Y., Zhu, P.-Q., Zhang, C.-L., & Jiang, W. (2018, August 13). Gut microbiota alterations in moderate to severe acne vulgaris patients. *Journal of Dermatology*, (45)10, 1166–1171. https://doi.org/10.1111/1346-8138.14586

13  Tan, J. K., & Bhate, K. (2015, July). A global perspective on the epidemiology of acne. *British Journal of Dermatology*, 172 Suppl 1:3–12. https://doi.org/10.1111/bjd.13462

14  Gether, L., Overgaard, L. K., Egeberg, A., & Thyssen, J. P. (2018, August). Incidence and prevalence of rosacea: A systematic review and meta-analysis. *British Journal of Dermatology*, 179(2), 282–289. https://doi.org/10.1111/bjd.16481

15  Salem et al. 2018.

16  Salem et al. 2018.

17  Saint-Criq, V., Lugo-Villarino, G., & Thomas, M. Dysbiosis, malnutrition, and enhanced gut-lung axis contribute to age-related respiratory diseases. *Ageing Research Reviews*, 66(101235). https://doi.org/10.1016/j.arr.2020.101235

18  Yeoh, Y. K., Zuo, T., Lui, G. C., Zhang, F., Liu, Q., Li, A. Y., Chung, A. C., Cheung, C. P., Tso, E. Y., Fung, K. S., Chan, V., Ling, L., Joynt, G., Hui, D. S., Chow, K. M., Ng, S., Li, T. C., Ng, R. W., Yip, T. C., ... Ng, S. C. (2021). Gut microbiota composition reflects disease severity and dysfunctional immune responses in patients with COVID-19. *Gut*, 70(4), 698–706. https://doi.org/10.1136/gutjnl-2020-323020

19  Özön, A. Ö., Karadaş, Ö., & Özge, A. (2016, September). Efficacy of diet restriction on migraines. *Noro Psikiyatri Arsivi*, 55(3), 233–237. https://doi.org/10.5152/npa.2016.15961

20  Gazerani, P. (2020, June 3). Migraine and diet. *Nutrients*, 12(6), 1658. https://doi.org/10.3390/nu12061658

21  Cámara-Lemarroy, C. R., Rodriguez-Gutierrez, R., Monreal-Robles, R., & Marfil-Rivera, A. (2016). Gastrointestinal disorders associated with migraine: A comprehensive review. *World Journal of Gastroenterology*, 22(36), 8149–8160. https://doi.org/10.3748/wjg.v22.i36.8149

22  Clapp, M., Aurora, N., Herrera, L., Bhatia, M., Wilen, E., & Wakefield, S. (2017, September 15). Gut microbiota's effect on mental health: The gut-brain axis. *Clinics and Practice, 7*(4), 987. https://doi.org:10.4081/cp.2017.987

23  Clapp et al. 2017.

24  Ritchie, H. (2018). Global mental health: Five key insights which emerge from the data. Our World in Data. Retrieved August 7, 2020, from https://ourworldindata.org/global-mental-health

25  Bravo, J. A., Forsythe, P., Chew, M. V., Escaravage, E., Savignac, H. M., Dinan, T. G., Bienenstock, J., & Cryan, J. F. (2011, September 20). Ingestion of *Lactobacillus* strain regulates emotional behavior and central GABA receptor expression in a mouse via the vagus nerve. *Proceedings of the National Academy of Sciences of the United States of America, 108*(38):16050–5. https://doi.org/10.1073/pnas.1102999108

26  Tillisch, K., Labus, J., Kilpatrick, L., Jiang, Z., Stains, J., Ebrat, B., Guyonnet, D., Legrain-Raspaud, S., Trotin, B., Naliboff, B., & Mayer, E. A. (2013). Consumption of fermented milk product with probiotic modulates brain activity. *Gastroenterology, 144*(7), 1394–1401.e14014. https://doi.org/10.1053/j.gastro.2013.02.043

27  Tillisch et al. 2013.

28  Allen, A. P., Hutch, W., Borre, Y. E., Kennedy, P. J., Temko, A., Boylan, G., Murphy, E., Cryan, J. F., Dinan, T. G., & Clarke, G. (2016, November 1). *Bifidobacterium longum* 1714 as a translational psychobiotic: Modulation of stress, electrophysiology and neurocognition in healthy volunteers. *Translational Psychiatry, 6*(11):e939. https://doi.org/10.1038/tp.2016.191

29  Huang, R., Wang, K., & Hu, J. (2016). Effect of probiotics on depression: A systematic review and meta-analysis of randomized controlled trials. *Nutrients, 8*(8), 483. https://doi.org/10.3390/nu8080483

30  Cerdó, T., Ruíz, A., Suárez, A., & Campoy, C. (2017, November 14). Probiotic, prebiotic, and brain development. *Nutrients 9*(11), 1247. https://doi.org:10.3390/nu9111247

31  Butler, M. I., Mörkl, S., Sandhu, K. V., Cryan, J. F., & Dinan, T. G. (2019) The gut microbiome and mental health: What should we tell our patients?: Le microbiote Intestinal et la Santé Mentale : que Devrions-Nous dire à nos Patients? *Canadian Journal of Psychiatry, 64*(11), 747–760. https://doi.org:10.1177/0706743719874168

32  Limbana, T., Khan, F., & Eskander, N. (2020, August 23). Gut microbiome and depression: How microbes affect the way we think. *Cureus, 12*(8), e9966. https://doi.org:10.7759/cureus.9966

33  Mayer, E. A., Knight, R., Mazmanian, S. K., Cryan, J. F., & Tillisch, K. (2014, November 12). Gut microbes and the brain: Paradigm shift in neuroscience. *Journal of Neuroscience, 34*(46), 15490–15496. https://doi.org:10.1523/JNEUROSCI.3299-14.2014

34  Tomova, A., Husarova, V., Lakatosova, S., Bakos, J., Vlkova, B., Babinska, K., & Ostatnikova, D. (2014, November 6). Gastrointestinal microbiota in children with autism in Slovakia. *Physiology & Behavior, 138*, 179–187. https://doi.org:10.1016/j.physbeh.2014.10.033

35  Li, Q., Han, Y., Dy, A. B. C., & Hagerman, R. J. (2017, April 28). The gut microbiota and autism spectrum disorders. *Front Cell Neuroscience, 11,* 120. https://doi.org:10.3389/fncel.2017.00120

36  Jiang, C., Li, G., Huang, P., Liu, Z., & Zhao, B. (2017). The gut microbiota and Alzheimer's disease. *Journal of Alzheimer's Disease, 58*(1), 1–15. https://doi.org:10.3233/JAD-161141

37  World Health Organization. (2021, September 2). *Dementia.* Newsroom/Fact sheets. https://www.who.int/news-room/fact-sheets/detail/dementia

38  Harach, T., Marungruang, N., Duthilleul, N., Cheatham, V., Mc Coy, K. D., Frisoni, G., Neher, J. J., Fåk, F., Jucker, M., Lasser, T., & Bolmont, T. (2017, February 8). Reduction of Abeta amyloid pathology in APPPS1 transgenic mice in the absence of gut microbiota. *Scientific Reports, 7*(41802). https://doi.org/10.1038/srep41802

39  National Institutes of Health. (2016, April 4). Gut microbes linked to rheumatoid arthritis. U. S. Department of Health & Human Services. Retrieved September 21, 2021, from https://www.nih.gov/news-events/nih-research-matters/gut-microbes-linked-rheumatoid-arthritis

40  Favazzo, L. J., Hendesi, H., Villani, D. A., Soniwala, S., Dar, Q. A., Schott, E. M., Gill, S. R., & Auscik, M. J. (2020). The gut microbiome-joint connection: Implications in osteoarthritis. *Current Opinion in Rheumatology, 32*(1), 92–101. https://doi.org/10.1097/BOR.0000000000000681

41  Szychlinska, M. A., Di Rosa, M., Castorina, A., Mobasheri, A., & Musumeci, G. (2019, January 12). A correlation between intestinal microbiota dysbiosis and osteoarthritis. *Heliyon, 5*(1), Article e01134. https://doi.org/10.1016/j.heliyon.2019.e01134

42  Bischoff, S. C., Barbara, G., Buurman, W., Ockhuizen, T., Schulzke, J.-D., Serino, M., Tilg, H., Watson, A., & Wells, J. M. (2014, November 18). Intestinal permeability—a new target for disease prevention and therapy. *BMC Gastroenterology, 14,* 189. https://doi.org/10.1186/s12876-014-0189-7

43  Hollander, D., & Kaunitz, J. D. (2020). The "leaky gut": Tight junctions but loose associations? *Digestive Diseases and Sciences, 65*(5), 1277–1287. https://doi.org/10.1007/s10620-019-05777-2

44  Farré, R., Fiorani, M., Abdu Rahiman, S., & Matteoli, G. (2020, April 23). Intestinal permeability, inflammation and the role of nutrients. *Nutrients, 12*(4), 1185. https://doi.org/10.3390/nu12041185

45  Krajmalnik-Brown, R., Ilhan, Z.-E., Kang, D. W., & DiBaise, J. K. (2012, April 27). Effects of gut microbes on nutrient absorption and energy regulation. *Nutrition in Clinical Practice, 27*(2), 201–214. https://doi.org:10.1177/0884533611436116

46  Boutagy, N. E., McMillan, R. P., Frisard, M. I., & Hulver, M. W. (2016, May). Metabolic endotoxemia with obesity: Is it real and is it relevant? *Biochimie, 124,* 11–20. https://doi.org/10.1016/j.biochi.2015.06.020

47  Pizzorno, J. (2014, December). Toxins from the gut. *Integrative Medicine, 13*(6), 8–11.

48  Pendyala, S., Walker, J. M., & Holt, P. R. (2012, May 1). A high-fat diet is associated with endotoxemia that originates from the gut. *Gastroenterology,* Article 142(5):1100–1101.e2. https://doi.org/10.1053/j.gastro.2012.01.034

49   Boutagy 2016.

50   Boutagy 2016.

## Chapter 3

1    Zhu, B., Wang, X., & Li, L. (2010). Human gut microbiome: The second genome of human body. *Protein & Cell, 1*(8), 718–725. https://doi.org/10.1007/s13238-010-0093-z

2    Clapp, M., Aurora, N., Herrera, L., Bhatia, M., Wilen, E., & Wakefield, S. (2017, September 15). Gut microbiota's effect on mental health: The gut-brain axis. *Clinics and Practice, 7*(4), 987. https://doi.org/10.4081/cp.2017.987

3    Wu, H.-J., & Wu, E. (2012, January). The role of gut microbiota in immune homeostasis and autoimmunity. *Gut Microbes 3*(1), 4–14. https://doi.org/10.4161/gmic.19320

4    Clemente, J. C., Manasson, J., & Scher, J. U. (2018, January 8). The role of the gut microbiome in systemic inflammatory disease. *Clinical Research Addition, 360,* j5145. https://doi.org/10.1136/bmj.j5145

5    Wastyk, H. C., Fragiadakis, G. K., Perelman, D., Dahan, D., Merrill, B. D., Yu, F. B., Topf, M., Gonzalez, C. G., Van Treuren, W., Han, S., Robinson, J. L., Elias, J. E., Sonnenburg, E. D., Gardner, C. D., & Sonnenburg, J. L. (2021, August 5). Gut-microbiota-targeted diets modulate human immune status. *Cell, 184*(16), 4137–4153.e14. https://doi.org/10.1016/j.cell.2021.06.019

6    Bamberger, C., Rossmeier, A., Lechner, K. Wu, L., Waldmann, E., Fischer, S., Stark, R. G., Altenhofer, J., Henze, K., & Parhofer, K. G. (2018, February 22). A walnut-enriched diet affects gut microbiome in healthy Caucasian subjects: A randomized, controlled trial. *Nutrients, 10*(2), 244. https://doi.org/10.3390/nu10020244.9

7    Maruvada, P., V. Leone, Kaplan, L. M., & Chang, E. B. (2017, November). The human microbiome and obesity: Moving beyond associations. *Cell Host & Microbe, 22*(5), 589–599. https://doi.org/10.1016/j.chom.2017.10.005

8    Saad, M. J. A., Santos, A., & Prada, P. O. (2016, July 1). Linking gut microbiota and inflammation to obesity and insulin resistance. *Physiology* (*Bethesda*), *31*(4), 283–293. https://doi.org/10.1152/physiol.00041.2015

9    Davis, C. D. (2016, July–August). The gut microbiome and its role in obesity. *Nutrition Today, 51*(4), 167–174. https://doi.org/10.1097/NT.0000000000000167

10   Menni, C., Jackson, M. A., Pallister, T., Steves, C. J., Spector, T. D., & Valdes, A. M. (2017, March). Gut microbiome diversity and high-fibre intake are related to lower long-term weight gain. *International Journal of Obesity, 41,* 1099–1105. https://doi.org/10.1038/ijo.2017.66

11   Ridaura, V. K., Faith, J. J., Rey, F. E., Cheng, J., Duncan, A. E., Kau, A. L., Griffin, N. W., Lombard, V., Henrissat, B., Bain, J. R., Muehlbauer, M. J., Ilkayeva, O., Semenkovich, C. F., Funai, K., Hayashi, D. K., Lyle, B. J., Martini, M. C., Ursell, L. K., Clemente, J. C., et al. (2013, September 6). Gut microbiota from twins discordant for obesity modulate metabolism in mice. *Science, 341*(6150):1241214. https://doi.org/10.1126/science.1241214

12   Ridaura et al. 2013.

13    Jiao, N., Baker, S. S., Nugent, C. A., Tsompana, M., Cai, L., Wang, Y., Buck, M. J., Genco., R. J., Baker, R. D., Zhu, R., & Zhu, L. (2018, April). Gut microbiome may contribute to insulin resistance and systemic inflammation in obese rodents: A meta-analysis. *Physiological Genomics, 50*(4), 244–254. https://doi.org/10.1152/physiolgenomics.00114.2017

14    Saad et al. 2016.

15    Magne, F., Gotteland, M., Gauthier, L., Zazueta, A., Pesoa, S., Navarrete, P., & Balamurugan, R. (2020, May 19). The *Firmicutes/Bacteroidetes* ratio: A relevant marker of gut dysbiosis in obese patients? *Nutrients, 12*(5), 1474. https://doi.org/10.3390/nu12051474

16    Baothman, O. A., Zamzami, M. A., Taher, I., Abubaker, J., & Abu-Farha, M. (2016). The role of gut microbiota in the development of obesity and diabetes. *Lipids in Health and Disease, 15*(108). https://doi.org/10.1186/s12944-016-0278-4

17    Baothman et al. 2016.

18    Jiao et al. 2018.

19    Most, J., Goossens, G. H., Reijnders, D., Canfora, E. E., Penders, J., & Blaak, E. E. (2017, June 16). Gut microbiota composition strongly correlates to peripheral insulin sensitivity in obese men but not in women. *Beneficial Microbes, 8*(4), 557–562. https://doi.org/10.3920/BM2016.0189

20    Saad et al. 2016.

## Chapter 4

1     Schnorr, S., Candela, M., Rampelli, S., Centanni, M., Consolandi, C., Basaglia, G., Turroni, S., Biagi, E., Peano, C., Severgnini, M., Fiori, J., Gotti, R., De Bellis, G., Luiselli, D., Brigidi, P., Mabulla, A., Marlowe, F., Henry, A. G., & Crittenden, A. N. (2014, April 15). Gut microbiome of the Hadza hunter-gatherers. *Nature Communications, 5*(3654). https://doi.org/10.1038/ncomms4654

2     Yong, E. (2021, May 3). *First look at the microbes of modern hunter-gatherers*. National Geographic. https://www.nationalgeographic.com/science/article/first-look-at-the-microbes-of-modern-hunter-gatherers

3     Centers for Disease Control. (2016, May 3). *CDC: 1 in 3 antibiotic prescriptions unnecessary* [Press release]. https://www.cdc.gov/media/releases/2016/p0503-unnecessary-prescriptions.html

4     Safrany, N., & Monnet, D. (2012, March). Antibiotics obtained without a prescription in Europe. *The Lancet Infectious Diseases*. https://doi.org/10.1016/S1473-3099(12)70017-8

5     Auta, A., Hadi, M.A., Oga, E., Adewuyi, E. O., Abdu-Aguye, S. N., Adeloye, D., Strickland-Hodge, B., & Morgan, D. J. (2018, July 5). Global access to antibiotics without prescription in community pharmacies: A systematic review and meta-analysis. *Journal of Infection*. https://doi.org/10.1016/j.jinf.2018.07.001

6     McFarland, L. V. (2008). Antibiotic-associated diarrhea: Epidemiology, trends and treatment. *Future Microbiology, 3*(5), 563–578. https://doi.org/10.2217/17460913.3.5.563

7   Conley, Z. C., Bodine, T. J., Chou, A., & Zechiedrich, L. (2018, March 1). Wicked: The untold story of ciprofloxacin. *PLoS Pathogens, 14*(3), e1006805. https://doi.org/10.1371/journal.ppat.1006805

8   Li, R., Wang, H., Shi, Q., Want, N., Zhang, Z., Xiong, C., Liu, J., Chen, Y., Jiang, L., & Jiang, Q. (2017, July 25). Effects of oral florfenicol and azithromycin on gut microbiota and adipogenesis in mice. *PLoS One, 12*(7), e0181690. https://doi.org/10.1371/journal.pone.0181690

9   Centers for Disease Control 2016.

10  ABIM Foundation. (2021, February 2). *Antibiotics for ear infections in children.* Choosing Wisely. Retrieved September 24, 2021, from https://www.choosingwisely.org/patient-resources/antibiotics-for-ear-infections-in-children/

11  Cox, L. M., & Blaser, M. J. (2015, March). Antibiotics in early life and obesity. *Nature Revies. Endocrinology, 11*(3), 182–190. https://doi.org/10.1038/nrendo.2014.210

12  Korpela, K., Salonen, A., Virta, L. J., Kekkonen, R. A., Forslund, K., Bork, P., & deVos, W. M. (2016, January 26). Intestinal microbiome is related to lifetime antibiotic use in Finnish pre-school children. *Nature Communications, 7,* 10410 https://doi.org/10.1038/ncomms10410

13  Spellberg, B., Bartlett, J. G., & Gilbert, D. N. (2013, January 24). The future of antibiotics and resistance. *New England Journal of Medicine, 368*(4), 299–302. https://doi.org10.1056/NEJMp1215093

14  Centers for Disease Control. (n.d.). *About antibiotic resistance.* Centers for Disease Control and Prevention. Retrieved September 25, 2021, from https://www.cdc.gov/drugresistance/about.html

15  Crinnion, W. J. Organic foods contain higher levels of certain nutrients, lower levels of pesticides, and may provide health benefits for the consumer. *Alternative Medicine Review: A Journal of Clinical Therapeutic, 15*(1), 4–12.

16  Daley, C. A, Abbott, A., Doyle, P.S., Nader, G. A., & Larson, S. (2020, March 10). A review of fatty acid profiles and antioxidant content in grass-fed and grain-fed beef. *Nutrition Journal, 9*(10). https://doi.org/10.1186/1475-2891-9-10

## Chapter 5

1   Derrien, M., Alvarez, A. S., & de Vos, W. M. (2019, December). The gut microbiota in the first decade of life. *Trends in microbiology, 27*(12), 997–1010. https://doi.org/10.1016/j.tim.2019.08.001

2   National Geographic Society. (n.d.). *Biodiversity.* National Geographic Society. Retrieved September 25, 2021, from https://education.nationalgeographic.org/resource/biodiversity

3   Agridigitale. (2021, April). *Soils host more than 25 percent of the world's biological diversity.* Agridigitale. Retrieved September 25, 2021, from https://agridigitale.top/art-soils_host_more_than_25_percent_of_the_world_s_biological_diversity.html

4   Herring, R., & Wirick, R. (Directors). (2018). *The need to grow* [Film]. Earth Conscious Films. https://www.earthconsciouslife.org/theneedtogrow

5    Sperber, A. D., Bangdiwala, S. I., Drossman, D. A., Ghoshal, U. C., Simren, M., Tack, J., Whitehead, W. E., Dumitrascu, D. L., Fang, X., Fukudo, S., Kellow, J, Okeke, E., Quigley, E. M. M., Schmulson, M., Whorwell, Pl, Archampong, T., Adibi, P., Andresen, V., Benninga, M. A., ... Palsson, O. S. (2020, April 12). Worldwide prevalence and burden of functional gastrointestinal disorders, results of Rome Foundation global study. *Journal of Gastroenterology*, 160(1), 99–114. https://doi.org/10.1053/j. gastro.2020.04.014

6    Grönroos, M., Parajuli, A., Laitinen, O.H.,Roslung, M. I., Vari, H. K., Hyöty, H., Puhakka, Riikka, & Sinkkonen, A.( 2019). Short-term direct contact with soil and plant materials leads to an immediate increase in diversity of skin microbiota. *MicrobiologyOpen*, 8(3), e00645. https://doi.org/10.1002/mbo3.645

7    Hunter, M. R., Gillespie, B. W., Chen, S. Y. (2019, April 4). Urban nature experiences reduce stress in the context of daily life based on salivary biomarkers. *Frontiers in Psychology*, 10, 722. https://doi.org/10.3389/fpsyg.2019.00722

8    Kadar, N., Romero, R., & Papp, Z. (2019, December). Ignaz Semmelweis: the "Savior of Mothers": On the 200th anniversary of his birth. *American Journal of Obstetrics & Gynecology*, 219(6), 519–522. https://doi.org/10.1016/j.ajog.2018.10.036

9    Gaulke, C. A., Barton, C. L., Proffitt, S., Tanguay, R. L., & Sharpton, T. J. (2016, May 18). Triclosan exposure is associated with rapid restructuring of the microbiome in adult zebrafish. *PLoS ONE*, 11(5): e0154632 https://doi.org/10.1371/journal. pone.0154632

10   Yang, H., Wang, W., Romano, K. A., Gu, M., Sanidad, K. Z., Kim, D., Yang, J., Schmidt, B., Panigrahy, D., Pei, R., Martin, D. A., Ozay, E. I., Wang, Y., Song, M., Bolling, B. W., Xiao, H., Minter, L. M., Yang, G.-Y., Xiu, Z., et al. (2018, May 30). A common antimicrobial additive increases colonic inflammation and colitis-associated colon tumorigenesis in mice. *Science Translational Medicine*, 10(443), eaan4116. https://doi. org/10.1126/scitranslmed.aan4116

11   Sanidad, K. Z., Xiao, H., & Zhang, G. (2019). Triclosan, a common antimicrobial ingredient, on gut microbiota and gut health. *Gut Microbes*, 10(3), 434–437. https://doi. org/10.1080/19490976.2018.1546521

12   Yu, J. J., Manus, M. B., Mueller, O., Windsor, S. C., Horvath, J. E., & Nunn, C. L. (2018, August 20). Antibacterial soap use impacts skin microbial communities in rural Madagascar. *PLoS One*, 13(8), e0199899. https://doi.org/10.1371/journal.pone.0199899

13   Segers, M. E., & Lebeer, S. (2014, August 29). Towards a better understanding of *Lactobacillus rhamnosus* GG—host interactions. *Microbial Cell Factories*, 13 Suppl 1, S7. https://doi.org/10.1186/1475-2859-13-S1-S7

14   Ejtahed, H. S., Hasani-Ranjbar, S., Siadat, S. D., & Larijani, B. (2020). The most important challenges ahead of microbiome pattern in the post era of the COVID-19 pandemic. *Journal of Diabetes and Metabolic Disorders*, 19(2), 1–3. https://doi. org/10.1007/s40200-020-00579-0

15   Alavanja, M. C. (2009). Introduction: pesticides use and exposure extensive worldwide. *Reviews on Environmental Health*, 24(4), 303–309. https://doi.org/10.1515/ reveh.2009.24.4.303

16    Bassil, K. L., Vakil, C., Sanborn, M., Cole, D. C., Kaur, J. S., Kerr, & K. J. (2007). Cancer health effects of pesticides: Systematic review. *Canadian Family Physician, 53*(10), 1704–1711.

17    Kamel, F., & Hoppin, J. A. (2004, June 1). Association of pesticide exposure with neurologic dysfunction and disease. *Environmental Health Perspectives, 112*(9), 950–958. https://doi.org/10.1289/ehp.7135

18    Ascherio, A., Chen, H., Weisskopf, M. G., O'Reilly, E., McCullough, M. L., Calle, E. E., Schwarzschild, M. A., & Thun, M. J. (2006, June 26). Pesticide exposure and risk for Parkinson's disease. *Annals of Neurology, 60*(2), 197–203. https://doi.org/10.1002/ana.20904

19    Nicolopoulou-Stamati, P., Maipas, S., Kotampasi, C., Stamatis, P., & Hens, L. (2016, July 18). Chemical pesticides and human health: The urgent need for a new concept in agriculture. *Frontiers in Public Health, 4*, 148. https://doi.org/10.3389/fpubh.2016.00148

20    Bretveld, R. W., Thomas, C. M., Scheepers, P. T., Zielhuis, G. A., & Roeleveld, N. (2006, May 31). Pesticide exposure: The hormonal function of the female reproductive system disrupted? *Reproductive Biology and Endocrinology, 4*, 30. https://doi.org/10.1186/1477-7827-4-30

21    Liu, J., & Schelar, E. (2012). Pesticide exposure and child neurodevelopment: Summary and implications. *Workplace Health & Safety, 60*(5), 235–243. https://doi.org/10.1177/216507991206000507

22    Tu, P., Chi, L., Bodnar, W., Zhang, Z., Gao, B., Bian, X., Stewart, J., Fry, R., & Lu, K. (2020, March 12). Gut microbiome toxicity: Connecting the environment and gut microbiome-associated diseases. *Toxics, 8*(1), 19. https://doi.org/10.3390/toxics8010019

23    Aristilde, L., Reed, M. L., Wilkes, R. A., Youngster, T., Kukuragya, M. A., Katz, V., & Sasaki, C. R. S. (2017, June 20). Glyphosate-induced specific and widespread perturbations in the metabolome of soil *Pseudomonas* species. *Frontiers in Environmental Science, 5*. https://doi.org/10.3389/fenvs.2017.00034

24    Istituto Ramazzini (n.d.). *How much glyphosate is used worldwide?* Global Glyphosate Study. https://glyphosatestudy.org/hrf_faq/how-much-glyphosate-is-used-worldwide/

25    Meftaul, I. M., Venkateswarlu, K., Dharmarajan, R., Annamalai, P., Asaduzzaman, M., Parven, A., & Megharaj, M. (2020). Controversies over human health and ecological impacts of glyphosate: Is it to be banned in modern agriculture? *Environmental Pollution, 263*, 114372. https://doi.org/10.1016/j.envpol.2020.114372

26    Organic Consumers Association. (2018, April 26). *Germany + 13 other countries say no to glyphosate: What about the U.S.?* Organic Consumers Association. Retrieved September 25, 2021, from https://www.organicconsumers.org/news/germany-13-other-countries-say-no-glyphosate-what-about-us

27    Carlson Law Firm. (2021, February 10). *Which countries and U.S. states are banning Roundup?* Carlson Law Firm. Retrieved September 25, 2021, from https://www.carlsonattorneys.com/news-and-update/banning-roundup

28  Walljasper, C. (Host). (2019, May 27). *Use of controversial weed killer glyphosate skyrockets on Midwest fields*. Harvest Public Media. https://www.harvestpublicmedia.org/post/use-controversial-weed-killer-glyphosate-skyrockets-midwest-fields

29  Agriculture in the Midwest. (n.d.). *Agriculture in the Midwest*. U.S. Department of Agriculture. Retrieved September 25, 2021, from https://www.climatehubs.usda.gov/hubs/midwest/topic/agriculture-midwest.

30  Centers for Disease Control and Prevention. (2021, September 27). *Adult obesity prevalence maps*. Centers for Disease Control and Prevention. Retrieved October 13, 2021, from https://www.cdc.gov/obesity/data/prevalence-maps.html

31  Carbajal, E. (2021, September 15). CDC: *Number of states with high obesity rates doubled since 2018*. Becker's Hospital Review. Retrieved October 13, 2021, from https://www.beckershospitalreview.com/public-health/cdc-number-of-states-with-high-obesity-rates-doubled-since-2018

32  Farmers Market Coalition. (2017, April 11). *Resources*. Farmers Market Coalition. Retrieved September 25, 2021, from https://farmersmarketcoalition.org/education/qanda/

33  Local Harvest. (n.d.). *Farmers' markets*. Local Harvest. Retrieved September 25, 2021, from https://www.localharvest.org/farmers-markets/

## Chapter 7

1  Flom, J. D., & Sicherer, S. H. (2019). Epidemiology of cow's milk allergy. *Nutrients*, 11(5), 1051. https://doi.org/10.3390/nu11051051

2  Vojdani, A., Turnpaugh, C., & Vojdani, E. (2018). Immune reactivity against a variety of mammalian milks and plant-based milk substitutes. *Journal of Dairy Research*, 85(3), 358–365. https://doi.org/10.1017/S0022029918000523

3  Chopra, A. (2020, March 11). *Milk alternatives*. Gastrointestinal Society. https://badgut.org/information-centre/health-nutrition/milk-alternatives/

4  Nikkhah Bodagh, M., Maleki, I., & Hekmatdoost, A. (2018). Ginger in gastrointestinal disorders: A systematic review of clinical trials. *Food Science and Nutrition*, 2(1), 96–108. https://doi.org/10.1002/fsn3.80

5  Dulbecco, P., & Savarino, V. (2013). Therapeutic potential of curcumin in digestive diseases. *World Journal of Gastroenterology*, 19(48), 9256–9270. https://doi.org/10.3748/wjg.v19.i48.9256

6  Hong, S. W., Chun, J., Park, S., Lee, H. J., Im, J. P., & Kim, J. S. (2018). Aloe vera is effective and safe in short-term treatment of irritable bowel syndrome: A systematic review and meta-analysis. *Journal of Neurogastroenterology Motility*, 24(4), 528–535. https://doi.org/10.5056/jnm18077

7  Endalamaw, F. D., & Chandravanshi, B. S. (2015). Levels of major and trace elements in fennel (*Foeniculum vulgari* Mill.) fruits cultivated in Ethiopia. *Springerplus*, 4(1), 5. https://doi.org/10.1186/2193-1801-4-5

8  Freed, D. L. J. (1999). Do dietary lectins cause disease? *BMJ*, 318(7190), 1023–1024. https://doi.org/10.1136/bmj.318.7190.1023

9   Pedre, V. (2021, August 6). What is the best diet for gut health? Happy Gut. https://www.happygutlife.com/what-is-the-best-diet-for-gut-health/

10  McFarlin, B. K., Henning, A. L., Bowman, E. M., Gary, M.A., & Carbajal, K. M. (2017). Oral spore-based probiotic supplementation was associated with reduced incidence of post-prandial dietary endotoxin, triglycerides, and disease risk biomarkers. *World Journal of Gastrointestinal Pathophysiology*, 8(3), 117–126. https://doi.org/10.4291/wjgp.v8.i3.117

11  Davis, C. D. (2016, July–August). The gut microbiome and its role in obesity. *Nutrition Today*, 51(4), 167–174. https://doi.org/10.1097/NT.0000000000000167

12  Davis 2016.

13  Voigt, R. M., Forsyth, C. B., Green, S. J., Engen, P. A., & Keshavarzian, A. (2016). Circadian rhythm and the gut microbiome. *International Review of Neurobiology, 131*, 193–205. https://doi.org/10.1016/bs.irn.2016.07.002

## Chapter 10

1   Porges, S. W. (2017). *The Pocket Guide to Polyvagal Theory: The Transformative Power of Feeling Safe*. W. W. Norton.

2   Porges 2017, 134–140.

3   Cani, P. D., & Knauf, C. (2016, May 27). How gut microbes talk to organs: The role of endocrine and nervous routes. *Molecular Metabolism*, 5(9), 743–752. https://doi.org/10.1016/j.molmet.2016.05.011

4   Bonaz, B., Sinniger, V., & Pellissier, S. (2017, November 2). The vagus nerve in the neuro-immune axis: Implications in the pathology of the gastrointestinal tract. *Frontiers in Immunology, 8*, 1452. https://doi.org/10.3389/fimmu.2017.01452

5   Pedre, V. (2021, July 9). *The secret to a healthy gut may actually be in your heart*. HAPPY GUT. Retrieved October 29, 2021, from https://www.happygutlife.com/the-secret-to-a-healthy-gut-may-actually-be-in-your-heart/

6   Physiopedia. (n.d.) *Vagus nerve*. Physiopedia. Retrieved October 14, 2021, from https://www.physio-pedia.com/Vagus_Nerve

7   Zhou, H., Liang, H., Li, Z. F., Xiang, H., Liu, W., & Li, J. G. (2013). Vagus nerve stimulation attenuates intestinal epithelial tight junctions disruption in endotoxemic mice through alpha7 nicotinic acetylcholine receptors. *Shock, 40*, 144–151. https://doi.org/10.1097/SHK.0b013e318299e9c0

8   Dattani, S., Ritchie, H., & Roser, M. (2021, August 20). *Mental health*. Our World in Data. Retrieved October 14, 2021, from https://ourworldindata.org/mental-health

9   Dattani 2021.

10  Pedre, V. (2021, June 18). *What traumatic brain injuries teach us about leaky gut + what you can do to heal today*. HAPPY GUT. Retrieved October 29, 2021, from https://www.happygutlife.com/what-traumatic-brain-injuries-teach-us-about-leaky-gut/

11  NES Health. (n.d.) "NES miHealth shows 93% effectiveness in outcome study." Retrieved September 30, 2022, from https://www.neshealth.com/nes-mihealth-outcome-study

12   McLaughlin, K. A., Rith-Najarian, L., Dirks, M. A., & Sheridan, M. A. (2015). Low vagal tone magnifies the association between psychosocial stress exposure and internalizing psychopathology in adolescents. *Journal of Clinical Child and Adolescent Psychology: The official journal for the Society of Clinical Child and Adolescent Psychology, American Psychological Association, Division 53*, 44(2), 314–328. https://doi.org/10.1080/1 5374416.2013.843464

13   Porges, S. W., Doussard-Roosevelt, J. A., & Maiti, A. K. (1994). Vagal tone and the physiological regulation of emotion. *Monographs of the Society for Research in Child Development*, 59(2/3), 167–186. https://doi.org/10.2307/1166144

14   Scott, B. G., & Weems, C.F. (2014). Resting vagal tone and vagal response to stress: associations with anxiety, aggression, and perceived anxiety control among youths. *Psychophysiology*, 51(8), 718–727. https://doi.org/10.1111/psyp.12218

15   Scott 2014.

16   Breit, S., Kupferberg, A., Rogler, G., & Hasler, G. (2018, March 13).Vagus nerve as modulator of the brain-gut axis in psychiatric and inflammatory disorders. *Frontiers in Psychiatry*, 9, 44. https://doi.org/10.3389/fpsyt.2018.0004

17   Tarn, J., Legg, S, Mitchell, S., Simon, B., & Ng, W.-F. (2019). The effects of noninvasive vagus nerve stimulation on fatigue and immune responses in patients with primary Sjögren's syndrome. *Neuromodulation*, 22(5), 580–585. https://doi.org/10.1111/ner.12879

18   Henssen, D. J. H. A., Derks, B., van Doorn, M., & Verhoogt, N. (2019). Vagus nerve stimulation for primary headache disorders: An anatomical review to explain a clinical phenomenon. *Cephalalgia: An International Journal of Headache*, 39(9), 1180–1194. https://doi.org/10.1177/0333102419833076

19   Yuan, H., & Silberstein, S. D. (2017). Vagus nerve stimulation and headache. *Headache*, 57 Suppl 1, 29–33. https://doi.org/10.1111/head.12721

20   Gottfried-Blackmore, A., Habtezion, A., & Nguyen, L. (2021). Noninvasive vagal nerve stimulation for gastroenterology pain disorders. *Pain Management*, 11(1), 89–96. https://doi.org/10.2217/pmt-2020-0067

21   Milovanovic, B., Filipovic, B., Mutavdzin, S., Zdravkovic, M., Gligorijevic, T., Paunovic, J., & Arsic, M. (2015, June 14). Cardiac autonomic dysfunction in patients with gastroesophageal reflux disease. *World Journal of Gastroenterology*, 21(22), 6982–6989. https://doi.org/10.3748/wjg.v21.i22.6982

22   Zhang, Y., Lu, T., Meng, Y., Alimujiang, M., Dong, Y., Li, S., Chen, Y., Yin, J., & Chen, J. D. Z. (2021). Auricular vagal nerve stimulation improves constipation by enhancing colon motility via the central-vagal efferent pathway in opioid-induced constipated rats. *Neuromodulation*. Advance online publication. https://doi.org/10.1111/ner.13406

23   Bugajski, A. J., Gil, K., Ziomber, A., Zurowski, D., Zaraska, W., & Thor, P. J. (2007). Effect of long-term vagal stimulation on food intake and body weight during diet induced obesity in rats. *Journal of Physiology and Pharmacology, 58 Suppl 1*, 5–12.

24   de Lartigue, G. (2016). Role of the vagus nerve in the development and treatment of diet-induced obesity. *Journal of Physiology*, 594(20), 5791–5815. https://doi.org/10.1113/ JP271538

25   Cleveland Clinic (n.d.). *Gastroparesis: Symptoms, causes, diagnosis & treatment.* Cleveland Clinic. Retrieved October 14, 2021, from https://my.clevelandclinic.org/health/diseases/15522-gastroparesis

26   International Foundation for Gastrointestinal Disorders. (2016, August 1). *Learn the facts about gastroparesis* [Press release]. https://iffgd.org/news/press-release/2016-0801-learn-the-facts-about-gastroparesis

27   National Institute of Diabetes and Digestive and Kidney Diseases. (n.d.). *Definition & facts for gastroparesis.* Retrieved October 29, 2021, from https://www.niddk.nih.gov/health-information/digestive-diseases/gastroparesis/definition-facts

28   *Gastroparesis.* (2020, October 14). Mayo Clinic. Retrieved October 14, 2021, from https://www.mayoclinic.org/diseases-conditions/gastroparesis/symptoms-causes/syc-20355787

29   Karkou, V., Aithal, S., Zubala, A., & Meekums, B. (2019, May 3). Effectiveness of dance movement therapy in the treatment of adults with depression: A systematic review with meta-analyses. *Frontiers in Psychology, 10,* 936.

30   Leyland, L. A, Spencer, B., Beale, N., Jones, T., & van Reekum, C. M. (2019, February 20). The effect of cycling on cognitive function and well-being in older adults. *PLoS One, 14*(2), Article e0211779. https://doi.org/10.1371/journal.pone.0211779

31   Ewert, A., & Chang, Y. (2018, May 17). Levels of nature and stress response. *Behavioral Sciences, 8*(5), 49. https://doi.org/10.3390/bs8050049

32   Goto, Y., Hayasaka, S., Kurihara, S., & Nakamura, Y. (2018, June 7). Physical and mental effects of bathing: A randomized intervention study. *Evidence-Based Complementary and Alternative Medicine: eCAM,* 9521086. https://doi.org/10.1155/2018/9521086

33   Laukkanen, T., Laukkanen, J. A,, & Kunutsor, S. K. (2018). Sauna bathing and risk of psychotic disorders: A prospective cohort study. *Medical Principals and Practice: International Journal of the Kuwait University, Health Science Centre, 27*(6), 562–569. https://doi.org/10.1159/000493392

34   Ma, X., Yue, Z. Q., Gong, Z. Q., Zhang, H., Duan, N. Y. Wei, G. X., & Li, Y. F. (2017 June 6). The effect of diaphragmatic breathing on attention, negative affect and stress in healthy adults. *Frontiers in Psychology, 8,* 874. https://doi.org/10.3389/fpsyg.2017.00874

35   Wang, Y., Kondo, T., Suzukamo, Y., Oouchida, Y., & Izumi, S. (2010). Vagal nerve regulation is essential for the increase in gastric motility in response to mild exercise. *Tohoku Journal of Experimental Medicine, 222*(2), 155–163. https://doi.org/10.1620/tjem.222.155

36   Forsythe, P., Bienenstock, J., & Kunze W. A. (2014). Vagal pathways for microbiome-brain-gut axis communication. *Advances in Experimental Medicine Biology, 817,* 115–133. https://doi.org/10.1007/978-1-4939-0897-4_5

37   Thoma, M. V., La Marca, R., Brönnimann, R., Finkel, L., Ehlert, U., & Nater, U. M. (2013, August 5). The effect of music on the human stress response. *PLoS One, 8*(8), e70156. https://doi.org/10.1371/journal.pone.0070156

38   Fancourt, D., Williamon. A., Carvalho, L.A., Steptoe, A., Dow, R., & Lewis, I. (2016, April 5). Singing modulates mood, stress, cortisol, cytokine and neuropeptide activity

in cancer patients and carers. *Ecancermedicalscience, 10*, 631. https://doi.org/10.3332/ecancer.2016.631

39    Porges 2017.

40    Fallis, J. (2017, January 21). *How to stimulate your vagus nerve for better mental health.* University of Ottawa. Retrieved October 15, 2021, from https://sass.uottawa.ca/sites/sass.uottawa.ca/files/how_to_stimulate_your_vagus_nerve_for_better_mental_health_1.pdf

41    Mäkinen, T. M., Mäntysaari, M., Pääkkönen, T., Jokelainen, J., Palinkas, L. A., Hassi, J., Leppäluoto, J., Tahvanainen, K., & Rintamäki, H. (2008). Autonomic nervous function during whole-body cold exposure before and after cold acclimation. *Aviation, Space, and Environmental Medicine. 79*(9), 875–882. https://doi.org/10.3357/asem.2235.2008

42    Jungmann, M., Vencatachellum, S., Van Ryckeghem, D., Vögele, C. (2018, October). Effects of cold stimulation on cardiac-vagal activation in healthy participants: Randomized controlled trial. *JMIR Formative Research 2*(2), e10257. https://doi.org/10.2196/10257

## Chapter 11

1    The Editors at Chopra.com. (2021, August 6). *How breathwork benefits the mind, body, and spirit.* Chopra. Retrieved November 30, 2021, from https://chopra.com/articles/how-breathwork-benefits-the-mind-body-and-spirit

2    Mirgain, S. A., Singles, J, & Hampton, A. (2016). *The power of breath: Diaphragmatic breathing.* U.S. Department of Veterans Affairs Whole Health Department. Retrieved December 6, 2021, from https://www.va.gov/WHOLEHEALTHLIBRARY/tools/diaphragmatic-breathing.asp

3    American Lung Association. (2018, June 20). *Five ways you might be breathing wrong.* Retrieved December 6, 2021, from https://www.lung.org/blog/you-might-be-breathing-wrong

4    O'Connor, K. M., Lucking, E. F., Cryan, J. F., & O'Halloran, K. D. (2020, July 11). Bugs, breathing and blood pressure: Microbiota-gut-brain axis signaling in cardiorespiratory control in health and disease. *Journal of Physiology, 598*(19), 4159–4179. https://doi.org/10.1113/JP280279

5    Cronkleton, E. (2019, April 29). *Breathwork basics, uses, and types.* Healthline. Retrieved November 30, 2021, from https://www.healthline.com/health/breathwork#uses

6    Mirgain 2016.

7    Hamasaki, H. (2020, October 15). Effects of diaphragmatic breathing on health: A narrative review. *Medicines, 7*(10), 65. https://doi.org/10.3390/medicines7100065

## Chapter 12

1    Ross, A. (2016, March 9). *How meditation went mainstream.* Time. https://time.com/4246928/meditation-history-buddhism

2    Mindworks Team. (n.d.) *A brief history of meditation.* Mindworks. https://mindworks.org/blog/history-origins-of-meditation/

3    Househam, A. M., Peterson, C. T., Mills, P. J., & Chopra, D. (2017) The effects of stress and meditation on the immune system, human microbiota, and epigenetics. *Advances in Mind-Body Medicine, 31*(4), 10–25. https://doi.org/10.3389/fnhum.2018.00315

4    National Center for Complementary and Integrative Health. (n.d.). *8 things to know about meditation for health.* U.S. Department of Health and Human Services. Retrieved January 12, 2022, from https://www.nccih.nih.gov/health/tips/things-to-know-about-meditation-for-health

5    National Institutes of Health. (2012, January). *Mindfulness matters.* U.S. Department of Health and Human Services. Retrieved June 2, 2020, from https://newsinhealth.nih.gov/2012/01/mindfulness-matters

6    Mindful Staff. (2020, July 8). *What is mindfulness?* Mindful. https://www.mindful.org/what-is-mindfulness/

7    National Center for Complementary and Integrative Health. *Meditation: In depth.* (2016, March). U.S. Department of Health and Human Services. Retrieved January 13, 2022, from National Center for Complementary and Integrative Health. https://www.nccih.nih.gov/health/meditation-in-depth

8    National Center for Complementary and Integrative Health 2016.

9    Goyal, M., Singh, S., Sibinga, E. M., Gould, N. F., Rowland-Seymour, A., Sharma, R., Berger, Z., Sleicher, D., Maron, D. D., Shihab, H. M., Ranasinghe, P. D., Linn, S., Saha, S., Bass, E. B., & Haythornthwaite, J. A. (2014) Meditation programs for psychological stress and well-being: A systematic review and meta-analysis. *JAMA Internal Medicine, 174*(3), 357–368. https://doi.org/10.1001/jamainternmed.2013.13018

10   Househam 2017.

11   Househam 2017.

12   Basso, J. C., McHale, A., Ende, V., Oberlin, D. J., & Suzuki, W. A. (2019). Brief, daily meditation enhances attention, memory, mood, and emotional regulation in non-experienced meditators. *Behavioural Brain Research, 356*, 208–220. https://doi.org/10.1016/j.bbr.2018.08.023

13   Norris, C. J., Creem, D., Hendler, R., & Kober, H. (2018). Brief mindfulness meditation improves attention in novices: Evidence from ERPs and moderation by neuroticism. *Frontiers in Human Neuroscience 12*, 315. https://doi.org/10.3389/fnhum.2018.00315

# INDEX

## V

vagal tone, 240–242
vaginal microbiome, 83
vagus nerve, 235–250
    dysfunction of, 3
    gut health affected by, 240
    location and function of, 235–239
    stimulating the, 241, 243–249
    underperformance of, 241–243
vascular diseases, 66
Vegetable Broth, 183
viral infections, 74
Virgin Passion Fruit Mojito, 181

## W

walnuts, 59
Warm Savory Breakfast Bowl, 176
weight
    and antibiotic use, 74, 75
    gaining, 48, 61–62, 65
    and gut microbiome, 60
    impact of gut flora on, 61–62
    obesity, 60–63
Western medicine/healthcare, 17–18, 26–27, 71
wheat, avoiding, 118
wheat intolerance, 44–45
wheat sensitivity, 44
white blood cells, 2
Wild-Caught Salmon Cakes, 201

## Y

yeast overgrowth, 20–23, 43
yoga, 247

## Z

Zen gut, 267–278
    guided meditations, 271–278
    how meditation helps the gut, 270–271
    meditation, 267–278
    mindfulness, 268–270

# ABOUT THE AUTHOR

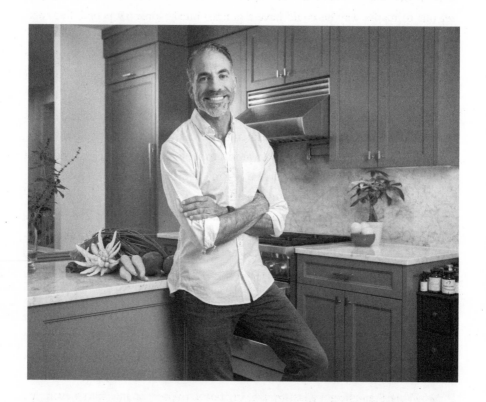

**Vincent Pedre, MD, is a board-certified internist and cutting-edge** Functional Medicine–certified doctor who is known as a wellness influencer, out-of-the-box thinker, medical sleuth, teacher, and engaging speaker. Recognized for his ability to connect with an audience, he has participated in innovative events such as Bouley Botanical's *The Chef & the Doctor* series, where food meets medicine; Tony Robbins's Life Mastery Program; and the Health Coach Institute Live, where he gave the keynote speech. He has crisscrossed the globe, teaching functional medicine to practitioners in Peru, Mexico, and Australia for the Institute for

Functional Medicine as part of their select bilingual international faculty team. And when not traveling, he serves a small group of motivated concierge patients who fulfill his desire to create deep, long-lasting relationships with those he cares for as a doctor, bringing the personal touch back to medicine.

Dr. Pedre's life and contributions have all been birthed from intention and grown through conscious choice. Not satisfied solely by the small impact he could have in the one-to-one clinic setting of his New York City private practice, he set out to map a way he could have a greater impact on how people live their lives—specifically, how they can be healthier.

However, between his dream and reality, many obstacles stood in the way. He was fraught with fears—the fear of public speaking, the fear of being in front of a camera, the fear that people wouldn't be interested in what he had to say. But he didn't let his fears get in the way of moving towards his life purpose: to help others live happier, healthier lives through the foundation of a healthy, happy gut.

Once he became clear that he wanted to help as many people as possible beyond the four walls of his clinic, he began a step-by-step plan to breathe life into his dreams. He needed writing experience, so in 2009 he started writing for the Food & Health blog of a health and wellness website called Ecomii.com. He attributes his brutal editor, Marie Oser, with shaping his ability to write about science in an easy-to-understand way for the layperson. This experience eventually helped him author his first book, *Happy Gut: The Cleansing Program to Help You Lose Weight, Gain Energy, and Eliminate Pain.*

He also needed to overcome his fear of public speaking, so he put himself in situations where he had to give talks and presentations. His first TV appearance was on *The Martha Stewart Show* in 2008. With no prior TV experience, it was a sink-or-swim moment, and yes—he swam! While fighting the fracking movement in New York State, he got a last-minute invitation to present at a charity event led by Mark Ruffalo because a blizzard had prevented the presenting doctor from driving into the city. In service of a higher purpose (protecting clean water for the millions in New York, New Jersey, and the Delaware River Basin), he couldn't say no. With only two hours to prepare, he had no time to work himself into a frenzy, discovering his ability to be an impromptu public speaker (even in the nerve-racking presence of such distinguished guests).

Dr. Pedre founded his private practice, Pedre Integrative Health, in 2004, the same year his son was born. Since then, he has manifested a multifaceted career as the adviser to two health-tech start-ups (one of which was recently valued at $450 million), an expert speaker for Orthomolecular Products, a nutraceutical consultant and brand spokesperson for NatureMD, and the founder and CEO of Happy Gut Life. An avid meditator, hiker, skier, and beach lover, he is also certified in yoga and medical acupuncture.

Dr. Pedre has also appeared on *Dr. Oz*, *Good Morning America*, *Fox News*, *The Early Show*, SiriusXM's *Doctor Radio*, and *Healthy Living* on ABC News, and has been interviewed on countless podcasts as well as quoted in online and print publications. He believes the gut is the gateway towards excellent wellness. Through his bestselling book, *Happy Gut*—featuring his proprietary "blueprint" for healing the gut, his Gut C.A.R.E. Program—he has helped thousands of people resolve their digestive and gut-related health issues. Dr. Pedre's own gut-healing journey served as inspiration for his unique approach, which includes balancing the gut microbiome, eating a gut-friendly diet, incorporating movement, following a non-toxic lifestyle, and practicing mindfulness for ultimate gut health and total body wellness. His newest book, *The GutSMART Protocol*, is the culmination of years of research and clinical experience as a functional gut health expert.